Transparent
Food Marketing

Transparent Food Marketing

A Clear Understanding of Food Marketing Terminology

Rachel E. Helwig

ISBN: 1514869861
ISBN 13: 9781514869864
Library of Congress Control Number: 2015911176
CreateSpace Independent Publishing Platform
North Charleston, South Carolina

TABLE OF CONTENTS

INTRODUCTION

I have worked within the grocery industry for over 14 years at many different levels, including buyer, so I have heard it all. I have been on the leading edge of trends and marketing ploys that have been used to increase sales. I believe in educating the public, and keeping them informed about what these terms really mean, instead of tricking people into buying something because of some buzz word. I have worked in multiple departments in stores, as well as in offices, making decisions about what to name a salad or how to rename a cut of meat to make it more appealing.

There has been a history of rebranding and remarketing in the grocery industry, in order to make something seem new that isn't, or to breathe new life into something that has slumped in sales. Although I find nothing wrong with that at face value, I feel that not enough has been done to inform the public as to what some words, terms, or commonly used phrases, actually mean. Nor has enough been done to educate the public on what barcodes are, and how they are used, and what they really mean.

The grocery industry and manufacturers are not the only ones guilty of creating this confusion. Often times, the internet can be just as guilty, if not more so. I am pained to have to admit that I have had to clarify some chain mail letters about "what things really mean" when it comes to UPC barcodes, PLUs, or even what certain terms mean according to an internet blogger. More than likely, someone had time on their hands, and an axe to grind, or they just wanted to see how many people they could confuse.

The goal of this book is to inform the average shopper about the vocabulary used in marketing grocery products, as well as what some of the key terms mean so that they are better able to make informed decisions about their purchases. It isn't to point a finger at manufacturers and retailers for their marketing practices, but rather make an informed consumer base. This consumer base may then be able to change some of these practices, instead of allowing retailers and manufacturers to make changes for them.

"Food for the body is not enough. There must be food for the soul."
– Dorothy Day

"Tell me what you eat, and I will tell you who you are."
– Jean Anthelme Brillat-Savarin

CHAPTER 1

TERMINOLOGY

There are a quite a few buzz words being tossed around that seem to carry a lot of clout in the grocery and food industries; but what do these words really mean? Below are some of the examples that pertain to food production, although there are others that are used to label products and make health claims, like gluten free or casein free. These are the terms that I feel have the most obfuscation associated with the actual meaning, as well as which organizations or logos can be used in good faith with the consumers purchasing these food goods.

It is important to understand the true meaning behind a word so that you do not become captivated by the newest, greatest, item that makes that claim or are swept up in the newest, latest, and greatest trends.

General Terms

- All Natural
- Organic
- GMO
- Non-GMO
- Hybridization
- Heirloom
- Fair-Trade
- Sustainability
- High-Fructose Corn Syrup

All Natural

A seemingly innocuous enough term that would make any shopper assume that the product may have been produced similarly to those that are certified organic, without having to jump through the hoops necessary to receive certification. However, according to the USDA "All Natural" simply means, "minimally processed", which leaves a lot to the imagination, and ultimately leaving no real regulations as to how this term can be used.

Simply looking at a grocery aisle can make this clearer to the consumer. Can a boxed dinner that is dehydrated, with added preservatives, and a shelf life that exceeds your own expected life span, really be "all natural"? This may be an extreme example with others that are available, such as Potato Chips or Frozen Fruit, but an "all natural" moniker means nothing as to how the product was grown, or even how it was processed and packaged. This also means nothing in the sustainability of the way the product was processed, or in the sustainability of the packaging used.

In poultry and meat processing, the use of "all natural" has the same meaning and does not refer to the type of housing or feed used on the animals during their rearing years. Although some have attempted to use "all natural" as a way to liken the item to Organic, it does not prohibit or prevent the use of GMO feed, Feed Lots, pesticides used on feed or grain, or any other process before the animal is slaughtered. The use of the term *All Natural does not* regulate the processes used during or after slaughter; the term simply means "minimally processed", and it regulates nothing in regard to what you are eating, or how it was raised or grown.

Organic

This seems straight forward enough. Organic: grown or raised without pesticides, antibiotics, hormones, or steroids, and only utilizing all natural fertilizers. By definition organic means it has not been genetically modified. This is the way everything was grown before the development of harsh pesticides and defoliants designed to kill weeds but keep crops growing. This term can be used in a variety of ways on different products. The USDA Organic seal can only be used on products that are certified through the USDA. Other organic markings may be used as long as the standards outlined in the labeling are not violated. For produce and livestock, there is only one marking for organic; for packaged products, however, there are many.

Packaged products may be labeled as USDA organic, or various levels of organic, from 100% organic to 75% organic. If 100% organic, this is explicitly stated on the label and in the round USDA Organic logo. Items that contain less than 100% organic; organic is listed in front of the ingredients that qualify as organic. Non-organic items are not required to be Non-GMO, or to be raised without any additives, pesticides, hormones, steroids or other possible toxins.

Organic labeling currently does not apply to seafood in the United States. There are foreign governing bodies that regulate organic certification for European fisheries. This certification is not identical to organic in the United States, and the USDA logo cannot be used on any fresh or processed seafood sold in the United States.

Why some farmers are so against Organic labeling?

It isn't that farmers are against growing foods organically, this couldn't be further from the truth. Organic demand is up, and has been, for the past 4 years, showing an 11% increase in 2013 over the previous year. As customer demand increases, so does the need to convert more farmland to organic farming. It isn't the practices used on organic farms either – farmers prefer using fewer chemicals, such as pesticides or herbicides, on crops as they know these can negatively impact surrounding farms and animals, or leech into the ground water supply and contaminate water used for human consumption, or for use on the crops.

So what is the problem? Payment. In order to receive organic certification, or the highly visible and instantly recognizable seal for USDA Organic, a farm must pay for inspections and pay for the certification.

However, this goes against laws enacted by our own federal government. 7 USC 2303: Prohibited Practices, Title 7 Agriculture, Chapter 56: Unfair Trade Practices Affecting Producers of Agricultural Products reads:

"It shall be unlawful for any handler knowingly to engage or permit any employee or agent to engage in the following practices:

a) To coerce any producer in the exercise of his right to join and belong to or to refrain from joining or belonging to an association of producers, or to refuse to deal with any producer because of the exercise of his rights to join and belong to such an association; or

b) To discriminate against any producer with respect to price, quantity, quality, or other terms of purchase, acquisition, or other handling of agricultural products because of his membership in or contract with an association of producers; or

c) To coerce or intimidate any producer to enter in, maintain, breach, cancel, or terminate a membership agreement or marketing contract with an association of producers or a contract with a handler; or

d) To pay or loan money, give any thing of value, or offer any other inducement or reward to a producer for refusing to or ceasing to belong to an association of producers; or

e) To make false reports about the finances, management, or activities of associations of producers or handlers; or

f) To conspire, combine, agree, or arrange with any other person to do, or aid or abet the doing of, any act made unlawful by this chapter"

If you read carefully through that lawful mumbo jumbo, you may have noticed that in in (a), it is unlawful to coerce farmers to have to belong to a particular organization, and that in (b) it is unlawful to discriminate against a farmer in any way due to membership or associations. However, in order to be certified as an Organic Farm and have the ability to have the highly recognizable "USDA Certified Organic" logo on your farmed goods, you must undergo USDA Organic Certification. This is a long process that takes years, as the soil must be tested and certified organic for two years. A conventional farm cannot convert overnight to organic, all trace elements of pesticides, herbicides and other non-organic chemicals must be absent from the soil in order to be certified.

While a USDA Certification can provide peace of mind to the consumer, and allows for a standard of practice for all farmers to follow, in addition to being healthier for humans and for the planet in the preservation of natural resources and the biodiversity that is present in organic farms, it is still a paid requirement to be a part of the association.

Non-certified organic farmers are faced with discrimination at markets due to the lack of certification, and often treated as conventional farmers and their product is treated as less valuable in the organic market. If a farmer uses organic practices they are able to claim that the product is organic, but they cannot use the USDA Organic seal on their product.

GMO

Genetically Modified Organism – GMO – this is a term that is often used out of context, or incorrectly, when discussing the growth of crops in agriculture. To clarify, this currently refers only to produce, as there is no GMO livestock in the market or in production. Implanting DNA into existing crops is a tedious process with extremely low success rates. Often times the plants are not viable with the location of the implanted DNA. A very low percentage of the GMO plants ever make it into full production, this has slowed the process in animals, due to the more complex nature of their DNA. This is surprisingly unsuccessful process with a very low percentage of those tried out in the lab making it to adulthood. There are a number of GMO items that are currently in production; corn, soy, sugar beets, alfalfa, canola, cotton, and papaya. Recently added have been potatoes and apples (a complete list can be found at www.nongmoproject.org). All GMO items can only exist through laboratory testing, as their genetic traits are selected or altered in the lab, at the DNA level. The most notorious of the GMO products is *RoundUp*. GMO ready products produced by Monsanto have glyphosate, the active ingredient in *RoundUp*, genetically spliced into corn and soybeans.

The idea behind GMO crops is to reduce the amount of sprayed pesticides used on the crops as they grow, while increasing the yields and ending world hunger. And much like a beauty pageant contestant's response, this is a lot of hot air and empty promises. There are many studies that show that the use of GMO crops have increased the amount of pesticides used, due to the adaptability of the pests that frequent these crops. There have also been concerns as the GMO pesticides in the DNA of the crop cannot be washed off, and have been certified for use through the FDA as antibiotics. This is a contributing factor in the creation of more superbugs that cannot be treated with normal antibiotics. Other studies look at yield of GMO crops and show that the yield is equal to, or less than, that of conventionally grown (non GMO, but with traditional pesticides), or organically grown produce. There are additional studies showing the negative effects of GMO raised livestock that include birth defects, problems with digestion, as well as other reported issues.

The purpose of this book isn't to turn everyone off of GMO; that research should be done independent of this book. Please keep in mind that studies should be looked at objectively as to who wrote the research, and the audience for which it was written. There are many studies on both sides of the issue that pander to the audience, and skew the data in favor of the author's preferred outcome.

Currently, there are no laws on the books that require labeling of GMO products as GMO, or containing GMO ingredients. However, some states have started to move forward on labeling as part of the "right to know" initiatives within those states.

You may have seen headlines on GMO Salmon. Recently, the FDA has been conducting studies on GMO or GE (Genetically Engineered) Salmon. This salmon was developed to grow 2-4 times faster than traditionally farmed salmon. The idea being to reduce the amount of time and resources needed to raise the salmon to maturity and provide increased turn over, and in turn, revenue, for the farmers. However, just like GMO plants, studies have shown that there are risks involved, so much so that most major retailers have refused to sell the salmon even if approved by the FDA. Just like plants, salmon is not required to be labeled as GMO when sold.

Non-GMO

The opposite of GMO, right? Well, kind of, but not really. Non-GMO is now a certification given to items that are conventionally grown and not organic, using pesticides. Unfortunately, due to the laws of nature and pollination, it is only through testing the crops that it can be determined if GMO items have not contaminated these conventionally grown crops.

There are a few third party non-profit organizations that certify items as free of GMO; including the *Non-GMO Project* (look for the butterfly). As with Organic, the farmers or producers of processed foods must pay for certification, or in this case testing, their product to ensure it is free of all GMO ingredients. Unlike some forms of Organic certification, there is only one level – completely GMO free. If an item is certified as Non-GMO, it is completely free of GMO. These products may have residual pesticides that can be washed off, but do not contain any additional, or modified, DNA from the items original form.

Using words like "real" does not mean that something is GMO free. For instance, carbonated beverage manufacturers have started to market versions of their beverages that contain "Real Sugar". This only references that they do not contain high fructose corn syrup, and instead use another sugar. This doesn't mean that the sugar used is GMO free. Only if the beverage is Non-GMO certified is it guaranteed to be GMO free – this is a concern, as sugar is very commonly GMO.

> *Made with Real Sugar does not mean that the sugar is GMO free. This simply indicates that high fructose corn syrup is not used. Only Non-GMO Certified or Organic products are guaranteed to be GMO free.*

How do GMO, Non-GMO and Organic Farms influence each other?

Let's just say, that GMO, Non-GMO and organic farms don't play well in the same sandbox, which has caused some problems with farmers. GMO farming uses pesticides and fertilizers in order to control pests and weeds and provide nutrients to the soil to increase growth.

Organic farming requires a payment to the USDA to ensure that the crops are in fact grown using Organic farming practices and are free from GMO contamination, while GMO farming is subsidized by the same organization. Organic farming doesn't use chemicals to inject nutrients into the soil, chemicals to rid the area of pests or chemicals to rid the area of weeds, so the overall operating costs are lower for organic farmers than GMO farmers. This isn't the reflection at the retailers as the Organic farmers pay for certification and testing of their crops, while GMO crops are subsidized to lower the operating costs and allow GMO farmers to sell their goods at market at more competitive retails.

GMO farming and organic farming cannot co-exist. In order for organic farming to be certified, it cannot have any GMO contamination. This happens through pollination via the wind or from insects; so additional space must exist to cut down on the risk of contamination. Organic farms and GMO farms cannot exist side by side. This same cross contamination exists with Non-GMO farms as well.

As a matter of fact, GMOs, because they are created in a lab can be copy written much like pharmaceuticals. The copyrighted DNA is then owned by the corporation that created the GMO in the lab. This company then sells seeds to farmers to grow the crops. These farmers, because they don't own the crops, are "renting" the seeds and cannot keep any crops to use for seed; but must rebuy the seeds each year. Additionally, if a farm is contaminated with GMO from cross pollination, the corporation that owns the rights to the GMO DNA can sue the farmers that are victims of nature – requiring the crops on the farmer's land to be destroyed, or fining the farmer for violating the corporation's ownership. In other words, the farmers are subject to charges of theft if GMO contamination is found on their farms.

This creates concerns, not only because the DNA itself is owned by large corporations, but because the growth of crops is a way to make a living. When that living is subject to suit due to natural processes like pollination from insects and wind it causes concern each time a GMO farm pops up, as the chances for contamination increase. These GMO farms also pose a threat due to concerns about how safe the chemicals used to destroy weeds and insects really are, both to the surrounding land and water, and how that will impact the surrounding farms that may not be using the same chemicals.

Cross contamination can be negative for GMO crops contaminated with non-GMO crops as well. With the absence or weakening of the DNA that was inserted in the lab, the effectiveness of the built in pesticide is weakened. This creates the need for excessive use of additional spray pesticides. This negative impact is faster than the natural adaptation of insects, and due to some plants having a weakened version of the pesticide due to the cross contamination with non-GMO plants, it can actually increase the rate of natural adaptation much like a vaccine prepares our immune systems for interaction with the full blown disease, as a weaker counterpart of the real thing.

Hybridization

This is what nature intended. This is how different items are produced through cross pollination; no need for a lab, or DNA manipulation. This is how Mendel bred pea plants to determine inheritance. Hybridization can be used to breed for specific traits, such as size, weight, muscle definition in livestock, or size of fruit, or ears of corn. It may also be used to combine two separate breeds to create a new one; this is often done to create new varieties of apples, an example of which is the Honeycrisp. Hybrids are generally created by forcing pollination of the plants in order to create a new variety, and then manipulating the future generations of that new variety to yield the best qualities. In the case of Honeycrisp, it was to ensure that the child generations would have crisp texture, thin skins that aren't overly bitter, and a sweet and juicy interior to the apple. This is generally done from heritage or heirloom varieties of the crop that the farmer wishes to hybridize – or an original species, form, or variety that could originally be found in the wild.

Through these natural processes, and through guided breeding or pollination, farmers can determine the results. They are also able to keep up with public demand for taste or yields in agriculture, while keeping out of the laboratories to do so.

Heirloom

This is a more recent buzzword, and has most commonly been used on "Heirloom Tomatoes". It can be found on other items, such as produce like Heirloom Pumpkins. The general term means that the plants are open-pollinated using classic practices. This means that forced pollination and GMO practices are not used to fertilize flowers on these plants; instead favoring wind, or bees, to pollinate the plants.

Over time, as transportation methods improved in speed, there became a higher demand for produce across the country and across the world. Methods were developed to breed produce that is more resilient to stacking and transportation practices allowing the produce to be distributed and transported very long distances year round to meet growing customer demand. In addition, this produce is also picked earlier in development, before fully ripe. This creates harder fruits or veggies that are able to withstand bruising unlike their ripe counterparts. These under ripe fruits or veggies are then gassed, or other methods are applied, to force ripening after getting closer to their final destination. Original heirloom varieties became less available in the market as they were not bred to withstand the long distances and the hardships of distribution. These heirloom varieties often have more flavor, tasting better than their traditional counterparts.

> *Refrigerated box cars were invented due to the popularity of Strawberries and the need for them year round on the eastern coast of the United States, driving the need for better systems of transportation and keeping produce fresh for long travels.*

Fair-Trade

This practice is based on equal treatment of farmers, distributers, and retailers to ensure that those trying to make a living are able to do so. Fair-Trade has been used for items that have historically been highly profitable for the retailers and distributers, but have not been as lucrative for the growers. Bananas, Chocolate, and Coffee are key examples of fair-trade products where farmers have historically not been paid their fair share of the profits from their goods.

Being Fair-Trade certified means that the products have been found to meet the guidelines of the non-profit that certifies them. The farmers are fairly compensated. Some consumers will note that fair-trade will likely increase the cost of the goods, but it also ensures that the farmers are able to make a decent living, keep their farms, seek proper medical care if needed, and provide money locally to help struggling economies.

Sustainability

You have probably heard the term "sustainable business" or "sustainable farming" or some other variation of the term in reference to the food chain, but what does it mean?

Everyone learned in school about the importance of crop rotation and keeping the crops diverse to ensure the crops are getting the highest amount of nutrients from the soil and, at the same time, providing nutrients to the soil for future crops. Sustainability refers to this type of practice; keeping the systems, or farms, diverse and productive. By rotating crops and keeping the crops that are planted diverse the soil remains productive. Planting the same crop year after year will void the soil of all useful nutrients for that crop and reduce the productivity of the soil, producing lower yields over time.

As a general term, this refers not only to the soil but to all aspects of the ecosystem in which the crops or livestock are grown and raised. This includes the impact of pesticides and fertilizers on local water supplies and on healthy insects such as bees – which are essential to the pollination of many species of plants.

If a crop or system is found to have a negative impact on any aspect of the ecosystem it isn't sustainable. Generally speaking, organically grown Non-GMO crops are the most sustainable as they use no pesticides, and only natural fertilizers, that pose no threat to local water supplies and actually attract good bugs within the ecosystem.

High-Fructose Corn Syrup

There is a lot of controversy behind the sweetener that is high-fructose corn syrup. This sweetener was developed when the cost of sugar increased, but large manufacturers still needed a less expensive sweetener. High-Fructose Corn Syrup was seen as the answer as corn was cheap and widely available. Many sugary items were sweetened with high-fructose corn syrup (HFCS) including sugary drinks and processed dinners.

What makes this so controversial? Recently, studies have been released that link high-fructose corn syrup to problems that range from cancer and leaky gut to obesity. Now, anything that contains high concentrations of sugar, of any kind, will contribute to obesity. This is amplified in individuals that have little to no self-control, or who consume a high percentage of calories in sugar each day.

The studies focus on the fact that high-fructose corn syrup has more complex bonds and is harder to digest than natural counter parts such as sucrose or fructose that are found in fruits and veggies. Natural sugar (cane sugar) is sucrose. Due to the bonds being more complex, they are actually harder for your body to break down and process naturally like it would sucrose, and your body ends up storing more as fat than would happen with natural sugars. Other concerns come from GMOs and other contaminants that are present in HFCS – there are pesticide residues, mercury and other contaminants that are not regulated or measured by the FDA, so impact on the population is not really understood.

High-fructose corn syrup is usually found in foods that are overly processed and contain minimum nutritional value. When you spot this, it is an indicator that the item isn't a health food, despite any other claims that may be present on the label. Beware, the food industry is aware of the apprehension of the public and the correlations of high fructose corn syrup and obesity in our society, and have started to market the HFCS under new names in order to get these by the average consumer.

Fructose and Fructose Syrup are now used instead of HFCS (High Fructose Corn Syrup). Fructose naturally occurs as a sugar in fruit, which is where the prefix "Fruct" originates, while "ose" means sugar. While fructose – as found in fruit and honey – is a natural compound, the fructose, fructose syrup or HFCS found on your food labels is generated in a lab in high concentrations in syrup form, to create a cheap sweetener for use in processed foods.

The danger may not be in the HFCS, but in the overall effect that the compound has on your body. Studies show that a diet that is high in sugar – natural, synthetic, or otherwise – can create food cravings and increase yeast and bad bacteria in your gut. This increase may lead to problems with your immune system, such as leaky gut, diabetes, arthritis, or chronic diarrhea or constipation.

High Fructose Corn Syrup is approximately 1.2 times sweeter than natural cane sugar, and in a highly concentrated syrup form, less is needed to get more "bang for your buck" in the food industry. No changes will be made on this compound unless customers speak with their money by refusing to buy anything made with HFCS as an ingredient.

Supplements

This is where things can become a little fuzzy. There are very few regulations that govern supplements; simply those below:

- Products that are manufactured and distributed must be safe
- Any claims made about products are not false or misleading
- The products must comply with the Federal Food, Drug and Cosmetic Act and FDA regulations in all other respects

What does this mean? Products that are sold as dietary supplements by either manufacturers or distributors are not required to go through FDA approval before being put on the market and labeled as dietary supplements. The manufacturer, distributor or firm responsible for the product must first make sure the above three requirements are met, but other regulations are not closely monitored.

This gap that exists between "what is food" and "what is a supplement" has created a miss understanding about claims that are made on products and how things are labeled. Dietary supplements will have a "Supplement Facts" label and foods will have a "Dietary Facts" label. The Supplement facts will list the active ingredients or the ingredients that are the marketing focus of the product such as Omega-3s, Calcium or other minerals and compounds. The remaining inert, or inactive binders, flavors, or fillers are listed beneath the chart with the active ingredients. What can be complicated about the label is that the serving sizes and % Daily Value (listed as %DV) is determined by the manufacturer, and sometimes followed within a particular industry between competitors, but is not based off of caloric intake and is not the same thing as a daily recommended value or DRV that is found on food labels.

Products manufactured and distributed must be safe

The FDA is out there to provide guidelines that promote safety – but there are always times when studies are altered or not conducted for long enough periods of time to ensure safety.

Any claims made about products are not false or misleading

In recent years this has become a problem, or rather, the problems have been rectified with fines and the products are pulled from the shelves due to misleading statements or false claims. In 2012 *5-Hour Energy* faced a class action lawsuit for false marketing claims on their product. This suit claimed that the whole advertising package, including displays and claims of "immediate energy", "no crash" along with pictures of being able to do activities such as mountain biking on steep courses were not experienced by clients. Eventually the law suit had to amend the original claim against *5-Hour Energy* because the claims from the manufacturer did not provide any physical harm to the plaintiffs. Ultimately claims were dismissed, but if you remember the original ads vs. those you will see today, there have been changes made. Namely, large disclaimers about what claims can and cannot do for your energy or that the "no crash" claim doesn't mean you won't experience a slump in your mind or body's energy but that you will not experience a "sugar crash" after consuming the product, as there is no added sugar. *5-Hour Energy* has also updated labels to include caffeine and other ingredients that were not previously listed.

In 2008 *Airborne* experienced a similar lawsuit for false claims in advertising their product. Originally marketed as the miracle product to boost your immune system for the frequent business traveler or teacher that is around germ infested children all day – this was the ticket to getting out of cold and flu season unscathed – and without a pocket full of used facial tissue. The inventor of Airborne was also a long time school teacher, which lent some credence to the claims, who would know better how to boost your immune system that someone that is at the front lines, a teacher or a doctor/nurse.

Airborne's main ingredient was vitamin C, which previous to the its release, through many different scientific studies was never found to boost immunity or increase resistance to diseases such as the common cold or the flu. After the suit was filed and went to trial, Airborne was forced to pay 23.3 million dollars in retribution for these false claims. Additional amendments have also been made to marketing campaigns as well as product packaging that make these claims.

Making a false or seemingly false claim can also be executed by asterisk or one of his close cousins. Watch for claims followed by symbols, these will likely state that the claim has not been evaluated by the FDA. This means that the FDA has not conducted an independent study to support the claims, or that there is no scientific basis for the claim. Some products will list studies or will share information from independent studies on their product packaging with claims if they are more reputable or in a field that has more years of study to support claims on packaging. Either way, beware of symbols located after statements and look for the meaning to make your own decisions about the reputability of the claims.

Recently there has been a surge of some products that have previously been marketed as Dietary Supplements being relabeled with a Food Facts Label. This, primarily, is due to the use of tax and food stamps. Food Stamps are federally regulated, which means that all states follow the same guidelines. The Tax that is applied to foods or nonfoods is dependent on the state regulations, but there are four categories that are used to classify an item.

1. Taxable & Food Stampable
2. Non-Taxable & Food Stampable
3. Taxable & Non-Food Stampable
4. Non-Taxable & Non-Food Stampable

As a general rule food is not taxed and nonfood items like bleach or a household sponge is taxed. "Food" is food Stampable, where the only requirement is that the item have a Nutritional Facts label and be regulated by the FDA – unfortunately there are not any requirements for the nutritional quality of that food. This leads to a large number of complaints about foods like cookies, potato chips and soda (pop) being purchased with food stamps and federal funding instead of the healthier alternatives. However, previous attempts by the FDA to redefine Food according to nutritional content or to classify some foods as "extravagant" have been too hard to implement or define in a way that can be easily executed, so there have not been any changes to the definition of food from the original definition.

Energy drink companies like Monster have changed from Supplement Facts labeling to Nutritional Facts labeling and gone under FDA regulation to avoid being taxed (as a food) as well as allowing the new "food" product to be purchased with food stamps.

Federal Food, Drug and Cosmetic Act and FDA regulations in all other respects

Perhaps the most vague and unclear requirement of a dietary supplement this basically states that the supplement industry cannot use ingredients that are banned in food and that sanitation, humane treatment, trade agreements and other regulations by the FDA must be followed.

This means that banned food additives like specific food colorings or lead must not be used in the production of a supplement. Basic sanitation and other federal requirements for the production of foods, drugs and cosmetics must also be followed to ensure the safety of those that choose to purchase the supplements.

CHAPTER 2

LABELING

There are three major ways in which a product can be labeled for easy scanning at the point of sale, for larger grocers or retailers that use scanners at the registers. They are PLUs, UPC barcodes, and price imbedded UPCs. UPC barcodes and price imbedded UPCs are discussed together as they are very similar in appearance, but are used on different items.

PLUs are used for bulk products as well as fresh produce. These help cashiers easily identify from the item what the correct code is, so that it is correctly processed at the point of sale for the guest. In addition, it is a universal system and allows growers to track a single sticker to place on the product before it is shipped out to a large distribution warehouse for delivery. After all, produce can come from all over the world, with large quantities shipping out of Guatemala, Argentina, Chile, Mexico, and Canada, in addition to many agricultural states in the US.

Country of origin is the last topic that is discussed, this is often very hard to understand; not only as a retailer trying to follow the rules set forth by the USDA, but also as a consumer trying to figure out why some things are labeled and others aren't. Hopefully, this is detailed enough to find out why, but unfortunately, not detailed enough to find out why the law is written the way it is.

<u>Labeling</u>

- UPC Barcodes
- PLUs
- Country Of Origin Labeling (COOL)
    - Produce
    - Meat (Beef, Lamb, Veal, Poultry, Pork)
    - Seafood

UPC Barcodes

There have been a lot of myths and chain letters that have been forwarded and distributed about Barcodes, and what all those numbers really mean. But, it isn't a conspiracy to keep the public in the dark about where product is grown, produced or processed. It is simply a code that is used by production companies, and can be scanned at any grocery, convenience, or party store, without causing any issues with store designated systems.

Obviously, our world economy has created more trade between states and countries than was present in the 1900's, when general stores had no need for barcodes. However, with grocers carrying well over 10,000 SKUs (different UPC Barcodes), it is important that these never duplicate to keep the items separate, charge the consumer the correct amount, and track inventories and orders at the store level.

Barcodes generally consist of 10-12 numbers. The first 5 numbers of the barcode are referred to as the Master UPC, and designate the manufacturer or business which owns the barcodes. Barcodes are regulated by a global organization, only one company can own a particular barcode. Barcodes can be purchased individually or in groups as large as may be needed by a manufacturer. Contrary to what you may have been told in a chain letter, nowhere in a barcode is there any designation for country of origin or processing.

Take another look at a barcode from a particular manufacturer; you will see a trend in the starting 5 digits, such as Nabisco, General Mills or Yoplait. All UPCs will start with the same 5 digit codes. For larger corporations, such as Kraft, there may be a number of different Master UPCs that exist in their lineup of products due to the companies that Kraft has purchased over the years. Over time, the UPCs may change to match the master UPC of the parent organization, or may remain the same master UPC of the company that was purchased. Whether the change is made is usually due to the number of products in the catalogue, or due to separate production facilities.

There are some barcodes that don't even have 10 digits, these are compressed barcodes. When scanned at a register, they will expand and add zeros to the center of the barcode to create a 10-12 digit barcode. POS (Point of Sale) software is built to do this automatically, and even these compressed barcodes follow the same rules as stated above. The next time you go shopping, you can check a 20 oz. bottle of pop, and some packages of gum. If the product is from the same manufacturer, you will notice that even the compressed barcode follows the same rules outlined above.

> UPC Barcodes are universal and refer to the parent company or manufacturer that produces the item with the barcode, not the country of production or the country where the ingredients originated.

There is a second type of barcode, a price imbedded or price driven UPC. Each code is generated at an individual store, and is unique for every retailer. There are some that are purchased regionally. These codes only appear on items that have a scale label. The UPC contains a 4-5 digit barcode for the scale, and then the price of the item. These bar-codes start with a 2, have a series of PLU numbers for the scale, and are followed by the price. These last digits in the barcode are generated by the scale, based on the quantity of units in a package, or the weight of the package for stores to label. There have been attempts made to make these PLUs more universal, so that all stores use the same code for NY Strip steaks, Boneless Skinless Chicken Breasts, or even pastries; this has been unsuccessful.

PLUs

You guessed it, these are universal too! This means that in our global economy, if you know a PLU for a banana, it is the same in the US as it is in France, 4011. PLU stands for Price Look Up code, and there is a standard listing for all products that are sold. PLUs are assigned to all existing produce. In addition, generic PLUs that can be used within a classification for any farmer raised or hybrid product that doesn't fall under the normal PLU number.

What you may not know is that there are currently three designa-tions for PLUs; Organic, Conventional, and GMO. Conventional is what you are used to seeing on produce; 4011 for bananas, 3107 for Navel Oranges, and so on. Organic uses the same 4 digit code that is used for conventional produce, but adds a prefix 9. Organic bananas become 94011 and organic navel organs become 93107. This is a universal pro-cess. Now for GMO. As previously mentioned, GMO items do not re-quire labeling to indicate the item is GMO. It was also mentioned that this labeling is universal, and designation is used within other countries including those within the European Union. For this a prefix 8 is used before the conventional 4 digit code. 84011 would stand for GMO ba-nanas and 83107 would stand for GMO navel oranges. In the United States, items that are GMO, and those that are conventional, are labeled in the same way. However, in other countries there is a designation be-tween the two.

Country of Origin Labeling (COOL)

Not every item needs to be labeled with the country of origin. Restaurants, farmers markets, and very small retailers are exempt from labeling, as are some items that only grow in specific regions. I will discuss the required items. The COOL regulation was put into place as a way to effectively trace food to the point of origin. This was done to minimize the length of a potential outbreak of salmonella, listeria or E. coli – this type of labeling makes finding the original point of origin easier, in order to reduce the number of people an outbreak like this would infect, or effect.

Eventually, the goal is to bring the COOL labeling to the individual farm or grower. This will make the labeling more effective for the reasons stated above.

What needs to be labeled?

Fish, shellfish, frozen and fresh fruits and vegetables, meat muscle cuts and ground beef (beef, pork, lamb, chicken & goat), as well as peanuts, pecans, macadamia nuts, and ginseng.

What is exempt?

Restaurants, cafeterias, lunch rooms, farmers markets, salad bars, delicatessens, and ready to eat food establishments are all exempt from declaring country of origin. There are also items within the grouping above, for those that require labeling, that can be considered exempt. This may seem confusing, and it is, but it boils down to two things:

1. If there is a change to the character of the item (remember your basic chemistry), if the item undergoes a chemical change, such as cooking, curing (like you would a ham), smoking or by changing the item's structure (like a fish stick), it is now exempt
2. If another food item is added to the mix; 2 or more food items mixed together no longer require country of origin labeling.

Mixing 2 or more food items is often called "further processing" in the food industry. This includes sausages, marinated or rubbed meats, stuffed meats, mixed fruits and veggies, or something as simple as a salt or pepper seasoning on a steak.

Things to consider

Sometimes, due to this regulation, the meat or deli departments within a retailer may be using meat that would not meet the standards for the meat department if the regulation were required. For instance, if the normal packaged meats are all prime cuts and all USA only, the kabobs that are considerably less per pound, could be from a different country of origin, or could be USDA Choice instead of prime. This allows retailers to save a little extra money. This is particularly true of some deli departments. When cooking meats that have more fat, such as those that are prime or choice, there is more shrinkage and loss of overall weight due to the water that is found in the fat tissue in the meat. As a result, some retailers will switch to USDA Choice from Prime, or will go from USDA Choice to Select, in order to save a little extra money. There is less loss due to shrinkage during the cooking process of these cuts, providing more value to some.

There are many honest retailers that are also doing their best to limit throw outs, and will utilize product from the meat departments keeping the standard across the board. Because the regulation does not require a country of origin to be stated when the product is cooked or has been further processed, further investigation is recommended on your part if this is of any particular importance to you.

Even if individual items at your local restaurant or the further processed items at your local grocer are not labeled with the country of origin, the vendors with which they are doing business are normally large enough to be required to have country of origin declared on the invoicing. This still allows some of the exempt businesses like restaurants, cafeterias, lunch rooms, or delicatessens to have the ability to trace the ingredients they are purchasing in case of an outbreak of any kind of contamination. Do not think that just because they are not required by law to declare the information directly to you means they do not have any ability to trace product or keep you safe?

What to look for?

There are acceptable and unacceptable ways to communicate the country of origin to the customers. Retailers must follow a strict list of guidelines that are designed to be clear and straightforward for the customer. This could be anything from placards, signs, labels, stickers, checkboxes, or other display methods. It is not ok to use flags to indicate the country of origin, unless the acceptable method is also followed. There are a lot of boring regulations regarding proper punctuation and abbreviations as this is a regulation set forth by the government, but there are some simple guidelines.

Even home delivery services and online retailers are required to state the country of origin as long as the product qualifies as non-exempt.

Produce

As previously stated, all fresh and frozen fruits and vegetables as well as peanuts, pecans, macadamia nuts, and ginseng are required to be labeled with Country of Origin.

Items that are clearly labeled by the farmer, manufacturer, or packer are exempt from additional signage. This could be a package for blueberries or a bag for oranges; or it could be a PLU sticker placed on the fruits or veggies before they are shipped out for distribution. Most retailers will not go through the trouble of labeling every single item through additional signage. It is hard to track country of origin through signage unless you are the one physically putting the product out. Only those items known not to have PLU stickers, and are unpackaged, are labeled with country of origin on signs – like jalapeno peppers. Items like bananas often have at least one sticker per bunch. This is considered adequate labeling, and counts as if each piece of fruit in the bunch were labeled. The display normally has enough available labels for customers to safely determine the country of origin.

Retailers are starting to focus more on "know who grows your food", and local marketing campaigns, to further the local economy for agriculture. Using local designations, such as state, city, or both, to communicate the country of origin is not enough. These displays and campaigns must also follow the federal guidelines and label the country – even if it is USA. Meats (Beef, Lamb, Veal, Poultry and Pork)
Covered commodities of meat muscle cuts, and ground meats for beef, pork, lamb, chicken, and goats require country of origin labeling. There are cuts that are exempt, such as femur bones, tails, tongue, neck bones, tripe, and cheek or skin. Beef patties are not required to have country of origin – these are not a "covered commodity", and are therefore exempt. Patties often contain binders or seasoning and are also exempt for that reason.

Labeling of meats is often more complicated than produce as the juvenile animals can walk around. There are many times farms that are close to borders of countries; an animal may be born in one country, wander into another, and then go to another to be slaughtered. In cases such as this, you may find multiple countries of origin on a single item. One common example is the USA, Canada, and Mexico. This can't happen with produce because trees and plants cannot get up and walk around.

Recent regulations have actually required, in addition to the country of origin being on the product, labels must show where it was slaughtered. Both where the animal was raised and where it was slaughtered must be clearly stated on the product. What does this mean?

1. Born or Raised
    a. Where the animal was born and reared before slaughter
    b. Or, if shipped to another country before slaughter, where did it spend its time before it was shipped away to slaughter
    c. "Hatched" can be used for chickens instead of born.
2. Slaughtered
    a. This is the point at which the animal is prepared for human consumption
    b. It is also common to see "harvested" instead of slaughtered, because that has a much fluffier, touchy, feely approach to the process.
    c. "Packaged" does not mean slaughtered, These can be two separate processes, and can lead to further contamination, if slaughtered in one location and packaged in another.
    d. "Processed" does not mean slaughtered. This refers to something along the lines of changing the already slaughtered chicken parts – like breasts – into nuggets or some other form.

When multiple countries of origin are required to be declared, the information must include where the animal was born, raised, and slaughtered. For instance:

- Born in Mexico, Raised & Slaughtered in USA
- Born in Canada, Raised in USA & Mexico, Slaughtered in USA

This is incredibly wordy, but allows for better tracking back to original farms should there be any outbreaks of diseases such as mad cow, E.coli, or listeria. Labeling is not done for food safety concerns until the two are linked, or when there is an outbreak of disease. This is done to easily track the animals back to the point of origin, to decrease the time contaminated product is available to consumers, increase the speed of recalls, or to allow customers to make choices based on the origin of the meats they are purchasing for consumption.

Many years ago, you may remember an outbreak of E.coli in fast food restaurants that ended in the death of many young children (due to their weakened immune systems). At the time there was no system in place, like that of the country of origin labeling, which could have easily traced and identified the source of the outbreak. This labeling is used to backtrack the path of the meats in order to determine where the contamination was introduced, what additional meats or restaurants may be affected, and therefore the risks to the general public.

These rules are also meant to prevent any contamination at the retailer level; meaning meats from different countries of origin, or points of slaughter, cannot be mixed into the same packages for sale. The products must be separated to reduce the risk of contamination from one source to the other. These products can exist in separate packages within the same display area, but cannot be packaged in the same container.

Some retailers may use a sign in the department near the display area instead of labeling each individual package. This is usually used for retailers that use only one place of birth, where it is raised, and where it is slaughtered for each species. You may see signs that say "All Chicken hatched and slaughtered in the USA" above or clearly displayed on a sign near the chicken found in the display cases. This labeling may also be found on stickers, scale labels, or on the packaging materials for the product in stores. The only regulation is, this must be clearly made available to the customers of retail stores.

Seafood

Seafood has always been a little trickier than other departments, or commodities, and has a history of obfuscation, or "pulling the wool over your eyes". This is clearly illustrated in the retail history of Orange Roughy. Originally known as "Slimehead", this species of fish was not selling well in the marketplace, obviously. However, this is a tender and delicious fish.

There was a marketing campaign in New Zealand to change the name to Orange Roughy, reflecting the orange scale color and the rocks near which it grows to maturity. This worked! It soon became the most valuable finfish species to be exported from New Zealand; so much so that it is now on the watch lists for overfishing. Orange Roughy is often illegally fished due to the small quotas provided by New Zealand to protect the species. The cold waters and depths at which this fish live cause it to mature slowly in order to reach sizes that are often used by retailers or restaurants. Orange Roughy isn't the only example of name changing and marketing campaigns that have been used to sell more seafood and increase exports. More examples, as well as specifics on species, alternative names, and preparation methods, can be found on www.seafoodsource.com/seafoodhandbook .

Regulatory agencies seem to think that country of origin labeling in Meats and Produce are too easy to follow, so they have come up with a completely different standard of labeling for seafood. In addition to listing the country, the method in which the seafood is raised is also listed on the product; either Farm Raised or Wild Caught. In addition, the country doesn't have to be the country in which the fish was raised or primarily lived, because this is a little more complicated than most COOL. I will go into a little more detail in an attempt to clarify.

Lake fish and Lobster are often found between the United States and Canada in our great lakes region, or off the coasts near Washington State, Alaska, or Maine. Most often Wild Caught fish have countries of origin listings that match the borders of the lakes or ocean that belong to that particular country. If the Lake Fish is caught closer to the Canadian coast, it is Canadian, if caught closer to Michigan, it is USA.

Fish or shellfish that are farm raised and then processed often only list the "last point of process" as the country of origin, and do not complete the entire chain. If a shrimp is raised in a farm in Indonesia, frozen for shipment in China, but bagged and processed in the USA, it can be labeled as USA. This becomes a little murky as product can be grown in countries that may be known for processes that are undesirable in other countries. There is no way to track, or follow, the point of origin based on the current labeling laws.

Labeling product with a country of origin based on processing does not apply to repacking. "Repacking" refers to the practice of taking a large packaged product, such as salmon fillets, from 20 pound packages for use in retailers or restaurants, to smaller 5-10 pound boxes. In this instance the licensed packer must label clearly the country of origin from the original box onto the boxes that are used for repacking.

Over the last 10 years, Antibiotics, Steroids, and Hormones have been hot topic buttons for discussions in regard to humans and their livestock. Superbugs and unwanted side effects, such as early onset puberty, early menopause, and zits, have all been attributed to, and discussed, when it comes to these commonly used compounds. However, you may not be aware of how these compounds are really being used.

Antibiotics are used for a number of reasons – prevention of illness, curing illness, and accelerating growth. Commonly referred to as "growth hormones", though not technically hormones, are antibiotics that have actually been known to cause accelerated growth. They are used most commonly in farm raised poultry or seafood, such as salmon. The same effect has been found to be true in pork and beef, though not to the same extent.

Steroids are a little more self-explanatory. It may be confusing as to why these would be used with the known negative consequences of prolonged use that has been observed in humans. These, simply put, are used to increase muscle development, or the overall yield of the livestock animals. Yield, in this example, simply means how much of a total weight of the animal can be utilized by the end user, or the shopper. The more muscle there is, and the less fat and bone, the more a farmer can get for an animal at slaughter. Though these effects can be reached through controlled breading, steroid use has been found to be faster and easier, with a more efficient result. Controlled breading programs, which pick the most appealing animals for reproduction to ensure these traits are passed on to future generations, take longer to establish and the results are not guaranteed. In other words, sometimes it is easier to cheat the system to get the desired end result without having to wait, and being more profitable in the process.

Hormones are chemical compounds that can naturally be found in an animal or have been synthetically produced to mimic an existing compound found in nature. Of the three, these may seem like the most innocent, as these compounds can be found in nature. However, the problem with hormones is they normally don't exist in large quantities, or they have been altered in a laboratory to last longer in the animal and could end up in your system as a result. Naturally occurring versions of the hormone would not last as long in the animal. The most widely known, and often times notorious hormone, is the bovine growth hormone, rBST. This is most commonly used in the beef industry to increase the size of the steer and its muscle capacity, as well as to increase milk production in some dairy cows. More recently, some retailers and manufacturers have started to advertise items as rBST free in order to get additional recognition.

In all cases, it is not a requirement that the labels at your local grocer, or even the menu at your local restaurant, label items as containing antibiotics, steroids or antibiotics. Most have started to label when products are free of these particular additives. It is important, however, to understand what that means based on the animal it is referencing.

CHAPTER 3

ANTIBIOTICS, STEROIDS & HORMONES

Recently there has been added attention to the subject of antibiotics, steroids and hormones as used in livestock. This is not only due to the controversial effect that the chemicals have on the livestock, and the resulting quality of life, but also because some of these synthetic chemicals can make it into the meat that is consumed by humans.

Even some common antibiotics that are used in humans have been found to have negative effects. This is carefully weighed by the doctor against the positive impact the compounds can have on your body, like curing a skin infection, which is necessary. These antibiotics were long ago, found to have similar effects on livestock, but had the added bonus of causing animals to grow faster and fatter. This allows famers to get the animals to slaughter in less time and utilize less resources in the process.

So what can be used, and why? This chapter will look at the uses of antibiotics, steroids and hormones according to the species of livestock. Each has regulations that differ due to metabolic rates as well as the time it takes in order for the animal to reach maturity.

Antibiotics, Steroids & Hormones

- Beef, Lamb, Veal and Pork
- Poultry
- Seafood
- Produce

Beef, Lamb, Veal and Pork

These animals often live longer than poultry, and as a result have more time to have these chemicals move out of their systems. It is important to look through the materials available to you from your grocer, restaurant, or on the internet, to verify claims made that the animal hasn't been provided any steroids, hormones, or antibiotics.

Specifically with antibiotics, there are often claims of "no longer using Human antibiotics", or "used sparingly". These often mean that breed specific antibiotics could still be utilized on the farm, such as one that was developed specifically for use on pigs. In the case of sparingly used antibiotics, it could mean that they are used only when an animal is sick. However, there are no real regulations on the verbiage used in marketing material in reference to these claims.

The most commonly used hormone among beef, lamb, veal and pork is rBST. This is the bovine growth hormone and has been linked to a number of health problems including ADHD, early onset puberty, and overall height and girth (meaning it could be contributing to America's obesity problem). It is not required that it be disclosed when this hormone is used. Recently, a large number of manufacturers have started to label product as rBST or RBST free in order to draw attention to the fact that it is not used in the meat or dairy products being purchased. If you are concerned about the use of this hormone in your daily diet, it is important to look for the rBST free claim either on the manufacturer's website, or on the product while shopping in stores. Without this claim, it is more likely than not rBST is being used at some point in the process of the livestock's growth.

Steroids can be legally used on beef, veal, lamb or pork items. These can make it into meat and dairy products processed from animals raised using them. These chemical compounds are most often used in humans to suppress the immune systems, which is why when steroids are used, most likely antibiotics are used. It is important to look for the claim of antibiotic free, as well as steroid free, if you are leery of these chemicals' use.

Poultry

Believe it or not, the USDA does not allow the use of Steroids or Hormones on poultry. Any poultry. Claims that products are steroid and hormone free means nothing, since no one is using them. But why claim this at all? Because rBST has gotten such a bad rap. Claiming to use milk sourced from rBST free cows is a marketing ploy, as the majority of manufacturers, large or small have discontinued the use of this particular hormone. This makes the item seem heathier than it is. As a consumer, you are more likely to buy an item that makes the claim than one that doesn't. But why can't hormones or steroids be used?

Poultry is processed at a very young age, only an average 49 days. The muscle tissue and metabolism of the animal aren't high enough to process the steroids and hormones out of the muscle tissue. If the USDA allowed the use of steroids or hormones, large quantities would remain in the muscle tissue of the poultry meats, and would make it into your system!

Antibiotics are widely used in poultry. Because the average life is only 49 days, farmers only want healthy poultry making it to market. These chemical compounds are often used to pre-emptively treat health issues before they can become a problem or spread. Antibiotics are also used as a "growth hormone" in poultry, and an effective one at that. You have likely walked the meat department at your local grocer, and looked at the boneless skinless breast that was larger than your closed fist, or even two of them, and wondered what created such a Franken-chicken. The likely answer is, unfortunately, antibiotics.

Seafood

Antibiotics are used preventatively, therapeutically, and as growth hormones in seafood. It is important to do research on your seafood to determine what is used. There are some responsible farmers that are using antibiotics only therapeutically, and not preventatively, or as growth hormones. These farmers are going to great lengths to get their message out there. These farmers only treat sick fish in isolated tanks so as not to contaminate the other fish in the population. They closely monitor the fish, keeping them out of processing until the antibiotics have fully made their way out of the animal's system, and therefore the affects will not reach the human that is consuming the flesh.

Organic fish will also be completely free of antibiotics. Unfortunately, there are no regulations governing an organic claim in the United States. There are, however, two foreign bodies that are reputable in registering an item as Organic. Natureland and the Organic Food Federation are currently used to certify or assist in standards of organic certification in Europe. The only seafood that is easily identifiable as being completely free of antibiotics, steroids, or hormones are those that are designated as wild caught. If the fish is not labeled as wild caught, it is important to ask questions; look for any further certification to ensure the seafood is free of antibiotics, steroids, or hormones.

Hormones and steroid use in seafood are not widely studied, but are used to increase growth and overall size of the seafood while cutting down on the amount of time the animal is raised before it is slaughtered. It is more common to find antibiotics used in seafood, though there is a lot of research money in the use of steroids and hormones to increase growth (decrease the amount of time it takes to "grow" a fully developed fish or shellfish in a farm) or to increase the yield (greatly increase the size of the fish or shellfish) with little increase in resources used to do so. As with antibiotics, the only way to be 100% sure is to ask a lot of questions, do the research, or buy Organic and Wild Caught products.

Often time chum or other processed fish byproducts are used to create feed for fish. It is important when looking into farm raised processes, to also look into the food that the farm is using. The fish itself may not be given antibiotics, steroids, or hormones, but the fish that was used to create the food pellets was given those chemical compounds. These pellets may be given to the fish, but they do not have to be declared because they are not given to the fish by traditional methods.

Did you know that Ruby Trout is actually a farm raised Rainbow Trout that was fed food additives, natural or synthetic? These additives are used in order to change the flesh color from a pink/orange color to a bright red color. This is not a different species.

> *Ruby Trout is not a separate species – This is Rainbow Trout fed color additives to change the color of the flesh.*

Do not be fooled. Wild Caught Ruby Trout does not exist.

Produce

Yes, even your produce can contain unwanted chemical compounds! Currently there isn't any produce that has hormones or steroids. However, GMO items do contain pesticides that cannot be removed or washed off before they are prepared – believe it or not, this pesticide is even registered with the FDA as an antibiotic.

The World Health Organization (WHO) has recently declared that this pesticide is cancerous, meaning that it has been proven to cause cancer. Some countries, such as Argentina, have even completely banned the use of this pesticide and all GMO crops. The reasons cited are damaged farmland, increased rates of cancer and birth defects, and lost income from farmers that have grown GMO crops for extended periods of time.

Organic certified produce are the only ones that can be easily identified as being GMO free. Some local farmers at farmers markets are using organic practices but cannot afford the certification. Retailers are now starting to focus more on local produce due to the reduced carbon footprint. The benefits are reduced resources used to ship, store, or even to force ripen product that is picked early and shipped long distances from farms, out of state or out of the country. This also helps to contribute positively to the local economic growth in the region, so win-win. When this happens, retailers will go out of their way to communicate the produce as being organically farmed, or being pesticide free. If you ever have any questions, make sure to ask your local retailer or farmers market. But, buyer beware, farmers markets can often times have large buying houses, or brokers that represent a large number of farms, that vary in growing practices. It is important you trust the person you are talking to, or ask follow up questions, in order to ensure you are comfortable with your purchase.

What about Vaccines?

Vaccines have recently gotten a bad rap due to pseudo-science and intentionally falsified studies. You may have heard some buzz on the internet that vaccines have led to an increase in the occurrence of autism. However, this study, and the studies used in the paper to support the findings were found to be false. Scientists whose studies were used within the paper have come out to state how false the findings were, and how a large amount of data was simply thrown out because it didn't fit the intended findings.

You may remember from elementary science that having a conclusion before conducting a study, and then only finding the results that support this conclusion, isn't real science. The risk of vaccines lies in the ingredients that can cause allergic reactions and for individuals that have compromised immune systems, not in those who are healthy, and vaccines do not create an increased risk for the occurrence of autism or other chronic illnesses.

Just like in humans, there are a number of diseases that pose a health risk for the animals and could potentially wipe out entire farm populations. These vaccines do not make it into the tissue of the fully grown animals and do not pose a health risk to the customers that buy or eat the meats. Vaccines must be continually used, even when the occurrence has dropped off or the disease will make a comeback, much like measles has in recent headlines.

A recent outbreak in pig populations has shown the impact of disease, and highly infectious diseases, among animal populations on farms. This virus, known as PEDv, wiped out 10% of the pig populations on US farms, increasing the cost of pork due to the shortages it caused. This particular virus was incredibly contagious and was found to be spread quickly from farm to farm by humans that came in contact with the virus. This could be from something as innocent as a trip to the grocery store or hardware store. If a farmer happened to get the virus on his shoes he could possibly transmit the virus to the pigs at his own farm. Both small farms, and large feed lots, were affected by this virus. A vaccine could have saved large quantities of the population, and will likely in the future, which would not only save a large number of animals from getting sick and dying, but also keep prices affordable.

CHAPTER 4

METHODS OF RAISING LIVESTOCK

O h the humanity! When it comes to raising livestock, there are a lot of popular buzzwords tossed around, in order to bring focus on the amount of effort a farmer must put into the general welfare of the animal, before it is ultimately slaughtered.

Thinking in terms of animal welfare was only recently brought to the public's attention with the work of Temple Grandin – an autistic savant. Grandin could "think like cows", and would walk through living quarters and slaughterhouses to provide insight into how much stress was being exhibited by the animals. The work of Temple Grandin, and a look into what her autism could contribute to the work of agriculture, was depicted in a major motion picture starring Clare Danes.

Other films have looked into the effect different forms of rearing and processing animals for consumption has on the animals' psyche, physical body including injury, as well as effects on the environment and future generations as a result of the carbon footprint. Some of these include "Food, Inc.", "Forks Over Knives" and "Fresh". All of these films look at the importance of proper diets in humans, and how the food chain plays into this diet. They also look into how our demand for an increase in less expensive foods in the United States has influenced how food is transported and processed, particularly livestock going from farm to table.

This chapter looks at the most common terms for livestock or by-products, and what these really mean in terms of humane treatment of animals. It will also look at what questions you may want to ask to ensure your purchases match your ethical standing on the humane treatment of animals. After all, to a marketing firm, sometimes close is close enough.

Methods of Raising Livestock

- Cage Free vs. Free Range
- Amish vs. Amish Raised
- Grass Fed vs. Grass Finished
- Humanely Raised

Cage Free vs. Free Range

These terms are thrown around in many commercials for eggs or poultry products, to make the product seem more humane for the chickens' but what does it all mean, and how does it affect the chicken? Some of this can be answered in a recent law enacted by the state of California, which may soon have your "grand slam" costing a whole lot more. California is the largest agricultural state in the United States, so they are often setting regulations that other states son follow.

According to this recent law hen houses have to make more room for each chicken that occupies the house inside the state of California, as well as all imported into the state of California - chickens and eggs must be reared in a hen house that has increased space for the chickens. This isn't a LOT of space, essentially taking the designated floor space per chicken from the size of an 8 ½ x 11 page of paper to that of an 8 ½ x 14 page of paper, allowing for a little more breathing room. However, this may open your eyes as to what kind of space, and the conditions, in which these animals are raised.

Both cage free and free range claims refer to the humane treatment of the animal as it is living its life up to when it is processed. Either as an egg producing chicken, and how the parents were living, or how the chicken lived before being processed into chicken nuggets.

Cage Free

In traditional chicken and egg producing farms, chickens are housed in battery cages and are limited in movement as well as the amount of space available for the bird. Now, this isn't a bleeding heart story about the inhumane treatment of animals. There are a couple of things to keep in mind when referencing chickens – chickens can easily be tricked. Tucking a chicken's head into its wing will hypnotize it into falling asleep, chickens do not often move, and may even stay put even when they have access to additional space. Chickens prefer warm and dark environments.

The battery cage system caters to the vampire like tendencies of chickens to prefer dark hot spaces. It also prevents movement in order to limit the chance of transmittable diseases, as much as can be done with little to no space between cages. The cage free system allows for the same amount of livable space as a battery cage system, but without the cage around the bird so the bird has the option to move around if it so desires.

This is a step up for humane practices of raising chickens and producing eggs. Some farmers and regulators claim that the cage free system actually produces more eggs, as the chickens are noticeably happier in the cage free environment, compared to those confined in a battery cage system.

Free Range

From the name you can probably guess the difference between a cage free and free range system. The Free range birds have access to the outdoors, or a fenced area outside the hen house. This system allows the birds to go in and out of the hen house as they please, and is used to encourage movement so that the birds do not become atrophied due to lack of movement inside the hen house.

What Makes Them The Same?

Often Free Range, Cage Free, and even the Battery Cage systems will use the same methods of slaughter when processing the birds for consumption. There are a number of ways that farmers will take their "mature" chickens to slaughter. I say mature in quotation marks because these birds are often taken to slaughter at about ½ their expected lifespan, when they are technically still juveniles.

Some houses will use concussion, while others will use a CO_2 gas that essentially puts the chicken into a coma, causing the chicken to die as a result of oxygen deprivation. Because retailers and restaurants are focused on selling you food to eat, this is often a topic that is skipped as it tends to make most people lose their appetites.

Why Not Allow for Outdoor Space Too?

Many farmers, or growers of chickens, will not allow the chickens to go outside for a number of reasons; such as avoiding any airborne contaminates. Chickens are susceptible to some of the same diseases that humans are, such as the avian flu, which is highly contagious. This particular strain of the flu is almost always lethal to chickens, although it presents only as a severe form of the flu when infecting humans. By allowing chickens outside, more are exposed to these factors. These chickens could then go back into the coop to infect the chickens that may not have ventured outside.

Amish vs. Amish Raised

This is a sore spot for me, as there are legitimate Amish companies that utilize the Amish farmers to raise and care for animals up until slaughter. There are companies that simply use Amish figures and logos to trick you into assuming that there is a special way in which the animals were raised; on big fluffy pillows to ensure the welfare of the animals. Now, even the Amish do not raise their livestock with big fluffy pillows, and they are raised without electricity. They are raised with excessive care and painstaking commitment to the welfare and integrity of true Amish products and services.

Amish

Many times when a label reads "Amish", it may look legitimate, but is probably not. These products usually show a horse and buggy, or an Amish family working hard on the farm, but do not use terminology such as "Raised".

These labels usually convey a healthy eating experience, as the Amish are raising their livestock without the use of Antibiotics, Steroids, or Hormones, and could generally be certified as organic based on the traditional practices of the people. However, the product that is labeled "Amish" is normally taking advantage of assumptions by the consumer in order to capitalize on extra sales. In this case, it is a "direct" misdirect on the behalf of the manufacturer. The product that is in the package is more than likely just as processed, full of antibiotics, steroids, hormones, or covered in pesticides, as the conventionally grown or GMO varieties of the same product.

Amish Raised

I am sorry to say that the waters are not much clearer – but equally muddied for this claim as they are for the Amish claim. As there are no federal guidelines to regulate this particular claim, anyone can make it and define it according to their company standard. But, there are companies out there that are being honest, and use this to convey the message that the product was raised in the Amish tradition, by those practicing the Amish faith.

Some companies make the appearance of having Amish farms raising animals, but are using the photos to sell more product. These companies have no integrity when it comes to labeling product with buggies, Amish farmers, or other common photos, to give the appearance that the animals were raised by Amish in the Amish tradition. These companies will often try to hide that the animals they have raised are conventionally farm raised, and may be missing claims that would legitimize the Amish claim, such as lacking an antibiotic free claim on the packaging. This can be a little harder to distinguish from the companies making the claim but also have no integrity. If you ask your local grocer, they should be able to answer questions regarding the legitimacy of the Amish claim.

From working with companies that are truly Amish – I have found they often go a little further out of their way to ensure the integrity of their final product than do conventional farmers. Miller Amish Chicken – a company out of Orland, Indiana is one of those companies. This company uses feed and bedding (chicken scratch) that has been tested to be free of asbestos, all vegetarian diets for the birds, cage free - not free range (free range exposes the animals to airborne contaminates, inclement weather and other risks that may become issues because no antibiotics are administered). These farmers also produce organically raised chickens without the use of antibiotics. The farms are certified by two separate third party organizations for humane treatment of animals, not only for the chickens, but all animals present on the farms where the chickens are raised. These standards exceed the standards set by Whole Foods whose standards are industry leading for retailers in the humane treatment of animals.

Don't be afraid to ask questions of your local grocer about brands they carry, and the claims that are made on the package, or even claims that the department employees know regarding that product that may not be on the package. The more informed you are, the more changes you are able to drive in the department with that almighty dollar – by buying, or not buying, what is carried, and providing the necessary feedback to the retailer.

Grass Fed vs. Grass Finished

This is confusing to anyone that isn't in the food industry. There are different types of grass fed processes that follow different guidelines in raising animals. What you have to realize is that traditionally raised livestock, particularly cattle, are free to roam across the plains until they get to a certain age of maturity. They are then sent to feed lots where they are essentially caged, much like the battery cage system used with poultry. Cattle are switched to grain for a number of reasons, it provides additional marbling, or fat swirling throughout the muscle tissue, and increases the overall weight including muscle development, to provide higher yields for the farmers selling the cattle to market.

This is important to the farmers raising the cattle, because the grain can increase the chances of having the cattle graded higher; such as Prime, or Choice, vs Select. This means that the marbling is more prevalent, and is more evenly disbursed throughout the muscle tissue. Standard Grass fed cattle will have much less fat, will often have a darker appearance to the muscle tissue (instead of a bright red color), and will have a slightly gamier taste. Farmers are looking for a higher grading as this means more profit, the higher the grading the more is paid per head at slaughter.

> All cattle start on a "grass fed" diet – do not fall victim to some of the Grass Fed claims.

Grass Fed

This indicates that the cattle were raised, primarily with a grass diet, and not grain. This does not mean that grass is the only diet that the animal received. Some grass fed products can actually be mostly grass fed, but finished in a feed lot. This is done for a couple reasons:

1. Some consumers want grass fed for health reasons, but hate the taste of 100% grass fed beef
2. Grass feeding cattle provides lower yields but still takes about the same resources to raise, such as water. It is in the best interest of the farmer to finish on grain in order to gain more profit from the animals

Some retailers can be a little deceptive on this claim. They will claim that all of their meat is from grass fed animals, as all cattle start on a grass fed diet. In order to be clear, ask your local retailer about the brands they carry. This is concerning because the grain finished meat does not provide same health benefits as the grass fed meats. Lower in Omega-3s, higher in cholesterol and fat, the grass fed meat provides better health alternatives to grain fed counterparts. If your morals do not align with the use of feed lots, or feeding an animal grain that would eat non-grains in the wild, then it is important that you do your homework to determine the true meaning of the claim.

Although a clear guidelines for claiming "grass fed" attributes seem to be lacking. There is a seal that can be placed to identify meats has having been raised completely on a grass fed diet. This is a USDA "process verified shield", stating that the beef meets the standards set by the USDA. Dairy cattle are certified as 100% grass fed in order to claim grass fed on dairy products like yogurt and milk through the *American Grassfed Association* (AGA). This organization looks at the diet and general welfare of the animals and ensures no diet supplements, like grain, antibiotics, hormones or steroids are used in rearing these animals. Just like the red meat, having a grass fed diet has positive health benefits to these byproducts. Increased omega-3, lower fat, and higher protein are some of these claims, though there are others.

Grass Finished

This is a term used to designate the diet of the animal toward the end of its life. This usually does not appear on the package, but may appear on the promotional materials found in your grocery store, or on the website of the manufacturer or packer. This term means the animal was never sent to a feed lot, and never had grain introduced to the diet. You may not be able to tell from the finished product in the store. If the muscle is red and bright, also known as the "Bloom", it is likely that the animal did not have a 100% grass fed diet. Grass fed beef tends to be dull in color with an almost brown hue (though still red). It is not the color we are used to seeing in the store as a regular shopper of red meats. This bright red color usually indicates that the animal spent some time in a feed lot eating grain in order to gain more moisture and fat and bring out the red coloration. The deceptive part of the bloom on meat is that it appears brighter, or more distinctly red, when there is fat (that white swirl in the meat), and the red also helps to hide additional fat!

I am not advocating that you shop for a darker meat because it will have a lower fat content if you are health conscious and looking for a healthier diet. Darker meat can also indicate that the meat has oxidized, or is starting to go bad. If you are concerned about the freshness or sanitary standing of a piece of meat, remember this – the meat should only appear to turn a darker red or a light brown color. Grey coloration, a green hue, or strange patterns on the meat (such as a thumb print on streak) will often indicate a sanitation or cross contamination issue where the meat was processed.

The bright color is attributed to the grain diet, and a 100% grass fed diet will leave the meat a muted red, almost burgundy, color and will often lead to premature oxidation; meaning the meat will start to turn to a brown color. This doesn't mean that the product is out of date or bad to eat, but that it has been in contact with oxygen. Grass fed products will often react faster to this process than animals exposed to a grain fed diet.

What is the big deal with grass fed?

The main reason grass fed beef is more popular than the grain fed alternative is that grass fed beef has more beneficial Omega-3 fatty acids, while the grain fed beef will have higher concentrations of Omega-6 fatty acids. Omega-3 and Omega-6 are both important to a healthy lifestyle, but what is more important is to establish a better balance between the two than can be found in the Standard American Diet.

Omega-3 fatty acid gets more coverage in news and studies, and this is because it is of vital importance to a lot of different functions in our bodies, particularly during early development and as we age. This fatty acid has been linked to an increase in brain volume and even reversing aspects of neurological aging. This is due to the fact that Omega-3 fatty acids make up about 8% of the brains weight and is a key building block in neurons. Omega-3 fatty acids are also linked to decreases in cardio-vascular disease as they assist in lowering cholesterol, keeping inflammatory responses in check and also play a role in curing diabetes and some forms of cancer. Omega-3, due to its important link to a healthy brain and neuron activity, has also been linked to a decrease in violent behavior and aggression (meaning those who are deficient in Omega-3 have been found to become more violent and aggressive), as well as helping to treat depression and other debilitating diseases with cognition, such as dementia and Alzheimer's.

Omega-6 receives less coverage, mainly because it is widely found in the current Standard American Diet as well as fast food chain foods, so there is no shortage or need for additional supplements and marketing to get your fill.

You need to eat foods that contain both Omega-3 and Omega-6 fatty acids because these are the two that are not produced by your own body. Many fatty acids are formed from your food for fuel, but these two fatty acids cannot be produced by the human body. Instead all quantities needed to function properly must be consumed through diet or additional supplements. The Standard American Diet is rich in Omega-6 fatty acids from sources like vegetable oils, vegetables, Canola Oil (rapeseed oil), Nuts, Cookies, Candies, other baked goods, cereals, popcorn, corn chips, tortilla chips, oil based dressings, and mayonnaise. All standard for the Standard American Diet (SAD).

As sources of Omega-6 fatty acids have become easier and easier to find and implement in our diets, the amount of Omega-3 fatty acids in our diets have declined. There are studies that suggest that the increases in obesity, diabetes and cardiovascular disease that are occurring in America are due to the decrease in Omega-3 fatty acids in our diets, and that balancing the Omega-3s back into the mix can help with these extremely expensive and potentially deadly diseases.

Good sources for Omega-3 fatty acids are fish, particularly Halibut, Herring, Mackerel, Oysters, Salmon, Sardines, Trout and Tuna. It is best that these are fresh, the cold temperatures from freezing and the hot temperatures from canning can break down the essential fatty acids, but if those are the only sources that is fine. Make sure that the fish is wild and not farm raised, or that the food used in a farm raised practice are rich with Omega-3. Traditional farming practices use foods that are good sources of Omega-6 fatty acids that greatly reduce the amount of Omega-3 in the farm raised sources while also increasing your intake of Oemga-6. Fish can produce Omega-3 naturally but must also get some from their diet to have the same quantities of the Omega-3 acid as the wild species.

Other sources can also be found. Some butters, eggs or juices as well as nut juices and yogurt are now fortified with Omega-3. Nuts are also a great source of Omega-3s. Flaxseed (ground so it is more easily digested, whole flaxseeds are difficult to digest and extract the essential amino acid), pumpkin seeds, and walnuts. Green leafy veggies are also a great source of Omega-3s. Brussels sprouts, kale, parsley, spinach, watercress and mint all provide a great source of Omega-3s along with other green leafy and fibrous vegetables. These veggies also provide a great source of other vitamins and minerals for your diet.

Oils that are traditionally plant based like vegetable oil, canola oil or peanut oil are generally high in Omega-6 with little to no Omega-3 fatty acids to add to your diet. Oils that are high in Omega-3 or that will help you to supplement your diet are primarily flaxseed oil or walnut oil. Another great substitute can be coconut-oil. Some vegetable oils are now fortified with Omega-3s to assist us in meeting our daily needs. Currently there is no daily recommended value based on any caloric intake suggested by the government. Most doctors promoting the consumption of additional supplements for getting Omega-3s or by changing your diet, recommend anywhere from 500-1,000 mg per day.

Cows that are eating a diet that is exclusively grass fed will have substantially higher quantities of Omega-3s from their leafy diet. Cows that are fed a grain based diet that promotes weight and fat to get to a Choice or Prime grading will have significantly higher quantities of Omega-6 fatty acids from the vegetable sources that they are consuming. So it isn't just what you eat, it is also what is being eaten by what you are eating that makes the biggest difference in your diet at the top of the food chain.

Humanely Raised

Humanely raised is also a claim with little meaning, like that of All Natural. There are no real guidelines defining what can qualify as humanely raised. There are regulations that farmers must meet in order to sell their product with USDA certification (which is a requirement to be sold in large grocers and retailers). The humane treatment of animals is dictated by the USDA. All manufacturers, processing plants, and farmers must meet these standards in order to sell their product at your local grocer. Processors and manufacturers that meet the USDA standard for humane and ethical treatment of animals can make this claim, and often do, though all processors and manufacturers are meeting the same minimum requirements set by the USDA.

Instead of looking for a generic claim regarding humane treatment, I recommend looking for a third party certification for the humane treatment, or research the company to find the standards they use. If you are looking for something above and beyond the manufacturer, retailer, or processing facility should be able to produce additional certification stating the additional measures they are taking to ensure the general welfare of the animals.

CHAPTER 5

GRADING

G rading often refers to the quality of a product, but there are different standards for every commodity. There are grading standards for eggs, feeder cattle, slaughter cattle, feeder pigs, slaughter lambs, yearlings and sheep, slaughter swine, vealers and slaughter calves, as well as for wool and mohair. That is a lot to go through, but this chapter will only outline the most common grades so that you are more educated on what these standards are. If you are looking for more information you can go to www.ams.usda.gov to look through more standards and regulations.

All of the regulations for grading are set by the USDA. Larger grocers, party stores, and retailers are required to sell product that has been certified or graded by the USDA. CSA (Community Supported Agriculture) groups are not required to put their product through the same regulatory standards, nor are small farmers' markets. With this, there is a chance some USDA sanitation or processing standards not being followed. Farmers that participate in these groups are often very passionate about their product, and work hard to ensure high quality. It is important when are purchasing from a farmers' market, or CSA, that you ask questions about the standards and about what the product may have been graded, if those qualities are important to you.

<u>Grading</u>

- Eggs
- Poultry
- Beef
- Ungraded
- Lamb, Veal
- Pork
- Seafood
- Honey

Eggs

While there are two primary grades for eggs used by the USDA found at your local retailer, AA and A, there is also a third, B. All grades are based on the condition and general appearance of the shell of the egg, in addition to what can be discerned about the contents as observed through the shell.

AA is the highest quality egg. These eggs are free from cracks, dirt, bubbles, and have the smallest air sack between the membrane surrounding the inner membrane (white and yolk), and the shell.

A grade eggs have almost identical standards for grading, but allow for a larger air sack between the inner membrane and the shell. It also allows for a slightly less defined yolk when looked at through candling light (originally this was done with candle light, and is now done with light bulbs that simulate the effect of candle light), compared to the AA grading. B grade eggs are not found in retailers as the eggs would not be pleasing to look at when cracked. The B grading still requires that the shell be free from cracks, but when looked at through candle light the yolk can be dark in color, flattened, or enlarged. The yolk can also show signs of germination (or chick growth), but cannot show blood when looked at through candle light. This grading can show serious defects that do not render it inedible, which is why this is not used in retail establishments – if you had one that matched this description, you probably wouldn't be buying eggs any time soon.

Keep in mind, this doesn't reference anything in terms of how the animal was raised, what the diet was, or how humanely the animals were treated while the eggs were harvested. This strictly looks at how the egg appears; including the internal structures as can be determined by candle light. This may or may not translate to a better eating experience, but the structure and integrity of the egg is closer to perfection with the AA grading.

Poultry

There are three grades for poultry, A, B and C. In most retailers only the A grade will show on packaged raw products, however, B may sometimes appear. This will explain the differences between the grades so you can better evaluate your purchases. Unlike eggs, the grade provided to poultry may reflect the general welfare and/or humane treatment of the animal leading to slaughter, this will be outlined below.

In addition to grading, there is a long list of terminology that determines proper naming of the animal and its parts; such as turkey, yearling turkey, chicken, ducks, geese, guineas, and pigeons, as well as sub categories for naming within each group. All of these terms are a bit much for anyone to take in all at once, but additional information can be found on www.ams.usda.gov if you are interested in this detail.

There are a couple of characteristics used to judge the grading for poultry, some dependent on weight. The basics are, deformities, skin coverage over the carcass, tears and cuts in the carcass, discoloration, broken bones, separation of the cartilage from the bones, and blood clots. There is additional information on standards for frozen poultry, and the effects of freezing on the carcass or parts, in addition to those already mentioned for fresh poultry.

There are a lot of guidelines, and reading the information from the USDA can be confusing as it applies to the grading. In addition to the weights and the associated percentages allowed at each weight, this is only an attempt to show the basic and most important aspects of each grade.

Grade A is free from deformities, has full or nearly full skin coverage, minimal tears and cuts to the carcass, minimal discoloration, no broken bones, no separation of the cartilage from the bones, and no blood clots. For Frozen Grade A poultry, the requirements are the same, but additionally, there can only be minor discoloration, due to the freezing process, on any part of the carcass.

Discoloration is normal, but remember that the discoloration should not look like large bruises on the carcass of the animal. Bruising that is dark purple in color means the animal was alive when the injury took place, and that there is a potential clot in the carcass. One or two shades darker than the skin or tissue color is completely normal due to regular processing of the animal.

Grade B quality product may have deformities such as dented or deformed bones, presence of small feathers on the carcass, a moderate covering of flesh or skin on the carcass, there may be broken bones or missing parts from the processing of the animal, moderate discoloration, some evidence of incomplete bleeding, light bruising, and may have slightly more damage. Grade B may also include a glossy appearance or lighter color due to freezing, than does the Grade A quality.

In some instances, the difference between Grade A and Grade B quality can reflect poorly on the manufacturer and cause concerns about humane treatment of the animal before slaughter. Stressed out animals, before slaughter, will often clench muscles causing more broken bones and discoloration of the skin and flesh. There have been some facilities that have worked hard to relieve the stress so that all processed birds can be of Grade A quality – these are the birds that get the most money at the market. Though Grade A does not guarantee the animal was treated well during its life, or even at the slaughter house, it does make it more likely because discoloration and broken bones are not allowed in Grade A.

Grade C refers to anything that does not qualify for A or B, but still meets a specific set of guidelines. Grade C is often only found in institutions, and even then rarely, and more likely to be used for feed for other animals. I will not go into further detail here, but as you can see from the regulations above, Grade C is not something you would want to eat.

Beef

You are probably familiar with the grading used on beef, as it has been all over commercials the past few years. These grades are USDA Prime, USDA Choice, and USDA Select. Any other designators, such as High Choice, Premium Choice, or Premium Select you may have seen in your supermarket or other retailers, are not regulated by the USDA. The retailer is required to define in their own words what these terms really mean and why they do not share the USDA designated grading. Sometimes this is done to expand a brand, or to try to separate a particular brand from everything else in the field. This has been done by packers and retailers alike. Packers have created two major brands of beef which fall under the USDA Choice and USDA Prime categories. These brands have further restrictions that make the standard harder to meet and allows the packers to reject more cattle, move them into other programs, or take the cattle into the branded program in order to drive prices up in the market. These two brands may sound familiar – Chairman's Reserve and Certified Angus Beef.

> Angus does not refer to a breed, or even a better eating experience; due to popular demand Angus has actually turned into a marketing ploy to sell more steaks and burgers from regular cattle.

Angus used to be defined as a breed of cattle such as Hereford, Holstein Friesian, or Brangus. The Angus breed was known for being all black, and as such, the black coloration was used to determine the qualifications into Angus programs. In science terms the designation went from genotypic (determined by the genes or breed of the animal) to phenotypic (how genes are expressed or the appearance of the animal and not the heritage of the animal). Now Angus refers to the black color covering all of the front of the animal with only about 25% of the portion of the steer with a color other than black. Angus is not a breed, or even a better eating experience; due to popular demand Angus has actually turned into a marketing ploy to sell more steaks and burgers from regular cattle.

The overall regulations that govern grading cattle is a whopping 18 pages long. Ultimately, the regulations come down to the correlation between the maturity of the animal before slaughter, marbling (fat between the muscles being evenly distributed throughout the muscle tissue creating a spotted texture much like that of marble), and the carcass quality grade. Carcass quality grade covers a large number of qualities, including the ossification of the bones or the discoloration on the internal marrow of the bone when the carcass is split for processing. There is a large series of other qualifications, but overall these are only important for a federal inspector at the processing plants and slaughter houses.

The main thing to remember is the age of the animal and the marbling, as these will determine the overall eating experience and consistent experience when buying particular meat products from a restaurant or grocer. Older muscle will be much thicker, making the individual muscles tougher when cooked. Marbling will create gaps between the muscle tissues and can increase the tenderness of an animal while also supplying flavor – fat is flavor!

For the best eating experience (juiciest and most tender, with the most flavor), you will need a young animal with a large amount of marbling. This is why USDA Prime is set at the highest standard and is the most expensive – it will also provide the most consistent eating experiences when purchased on a regular basis.

USDA Prime is the highest ranking. All USDA Prime, USDA Choice, and USDA Select follow the same general guidelines for age. The grade decreases as less marbling is present in the carcass. The only real difference between the three is the amount of fat – if you are on a low fat diet, or are concerned about the intake of fats from red meats, it is important you chose USDA Select. In addition to the grade, it is important that you chose cuts from the animal that have the lowest overall naturally occurring fats.

Studies have been done where fat is removed from muscle and fat from pork or lamb is added to just the beef muscle – the result was beef that tasted like the pork or lamb; the fat is what gave it flavor.
Fat is Flavor!

In addition to the USDA Prime, USDA Choice, and USDA Select designations, there is also a separate designation commonly used on the ground beef in your local grocer. You may see Sirloin, Round, Chuck, or percentages such as 80/20 or 72/28. The designations Sirloin, Round, and Chuck refer to the area of the animal that the ground beef comes from, but is only guaranteed to come from that area if it is marked as "Certified"; such as Certified Chuck or Certified Sirloin. The percentages refer to the percent of Lean Muscle to Fat in the ground meat. For certified programs you may see a Certified Chuck label along with the corresponding percentages. In this case, the fat is not tested but is naturally occurring at that percentage because it comes from those specific muscles in the animal.

Chuck has the most naturally occurring fat and is often used in slow roasting techniques. Chuck is not recommended for high heat, such as a steak, but makes great burgers due to the additional fat and flavor. Sirloin is the leanest of the three and does not work well for the slow roasting techniques, but cooks better at high heat for short periods of time for best results. Round is somewhere in the middle, and can often be substituted for either if you are looking for a leaner diet or want a little more flavor than Sirloin would provide.

You may find leaner, 98% lean or 96% lean – these are not certified to come from any particular cut, so if that is important for dietary or religious reasons you may want to avoid these. These mixes usually come from a combination of Round, Chuck, and Sirloin. The additional fat is leaned out, or cut off of, the pieces of meat before they are ground, until the final mix is as lean as needed to meet the percentages on the package or signs.

Ungraded

It may seem strange to talk about ungraded product in a section that is about grading, but sometimes retailers or marketing moguls will try to sell something that is ungraded. These products are presented as if they are a cheaper or more affordable version identical to the USDA Choice or USDA Prime equivalent. The thing is, it is not.

In order for a carcass of beef to qualify as ungraded, or to no longer qualify for USDA Choice (or any of the other gradings) the problem isn't marbling, but age. Remember that the older the beef the tougher it is. These are often advertised as a "Slow Roasting" version of the graded equivalent, or it is recommended to be best in the slow cooker. There are even times when it is explicitly mentioned that the cut is not recommended for BBQ, or to not cook on high heat for a short time, like you normally would as a steak.

The ungraded beef usually becomes more common when the market is just right; when milk is inexpensive, and beef prices are high. Raising cattle costs about the same, if it is dairy or raised for the beef market. This means that farmers are getting a higher return when the animals are slaughtered than when they are raised for dairy. Because the dairy cows are older they will no longer qualify for the USDA Prime, Choice, or Select rankings so they are slaughtered and then marked as ungraded or will not have the USDA Prime, Choice or Select stamps on the outside of the package. Some retailers even go so far as to state that the animal is grass fed as most dairy cows have more grass in their diet, or are on grass longer than cows, who are fattened on feed lots for slaughter.

Lamb

Lamb, sold at retail, only has two grades, USDA Prime and USDA Choice. A very large percentage get the USDA Choice grading with very, very little ever getting the USDA Prime designation. Like beef, this is primarily determined based on factors of maturity, marbling (referred to in the charts and records as flank fat, or the amount of fat found across the back and marbled throughout the muscle tissue) and quality. Quality refers to the overall appearance and development of the animal, meaning without deformities or defects.

Like with beef, the higher the flank fat or marbling the higher the grade. USDA Prime is the highest, then USDA Choice. There are grades below this, but you will not find these in your local retailer.

Veal

Again, like beef and lamb, the grading is determined according to age or maturity, the marbling, referred to in documentation as feathering, flank fat streaking, as well as the quality of the carcass. Age is generally determined based on the coloration of the muscle tissue. Veal will have greyish pink lean tissue that is velvety in texture, the fat will be soft. Calves will have tissue that is moderately red, losing the pink color, with slightly harder fat.

USDA Prime and USDA Choice are again used in Veal. However, unlike Lamb or mature beef, there are high point regulations with USDA Prime, and the animal may have too much fat to qualify for

USDA Prime. Like Beef and Lamb, the qualifiers are quality, marbling, and age.

Fat in older animals, like those in the beef category, is hard. In the meat industry this is often referred to as "Bark" – because if the fat covering a particular cut of meat is thick enough, more than 1 inch, it can actually feel like bark and make the meat feel as if it is frozen, even when it is not, simply because of how hard the fat feels.

> *Fat in mature beef carcasses or cuts is often referred to as "Bark" – if the fat is thick enough the beef may seem frozen to the touch because of how hard the fat feels.*

Younger animals do not have as much fat, or fat that is as dense. The fat will often be much softer and easily manipulated when touched. There are times when a retailer will try to pass off an older animal as veal or as a calf. You can easily test this by touching the fat through the wrapping material; if it is hard, the animal was not young at the time of slaughter. The animal was older and a gas compound was added before packaging to change the coloration to look more like veal or calf, or to reduce the bright red color common to the mature beef.

Pork

Pork does not use a familiar grading system, such as USDA Prime, USDA Choice, Grade A, or Grade B. Instead, there is a whole new grading process for the pork industry. This is U.S. No. 1 through U.S. No. 4. However, this grading is normally never found in a retail or restaurant environment, because as a consumer, no one knows what this really means.

I will not go into the details for every ranking, as these do not appear anywhere for you to investigate further, but ultimately it refers to some of the same qualities used in grading other species. Quality, fat - and newly - yield. Yield refers to how much certain cuts, which amount to over 40% of the total weight of the anima, will yield in relation to fat vs. muscle, or how lean this portion of the animal ends up being. The leaner the portion the higher the yield, as more muscle will be utilized and more of the fat will be marbled evenly throughout the muscle tissue instead of creating a "fat cap", or thick layer of fat around the outside of the muscle tissue, which cannot be utilized by the retailer, restaurateur, or customer.

Seafood

Seafood does not follow the same standards and guidelines that exist for other species; instead, they play by their own rules. Most of this is in reference to sizing. Sizing is most common in shellfish. Common indicators will be two numbers with a slash followed by count, such as 10/15 CT or 26/30 CT. With or without the count, this is in reference to the number of the item that equal a pound. A 26/30 Count Shrimp will have 26-30 shrimp in a pound, these are about average in size. The smaller the numbers the larger the shrimp will be, or the higher the count the smaller the shrimp. This is used to determine if it is appropriate to use the shrimp in a particular dish, smaller shrimp being most commonly used in salads and other dishes, while the larger shrimp are used in cocktails. A 26/30 count shrimp will often be recommended by the retailer to use in shrimp cocktail at home; in restaurants you will often find larger shrimp for this dish.

Other designations may be designated with U and then a number, such as U-10. This is similar to the designation that is used on shrimp. U means under, and the number indicates that the number indicated, or less, will make one pound. This is most common for scallops in a grocery retail environment.

There are no other quality or grading standards for seafood that indicate a particular fillet of salmon is superior to another. This is purely subjective, but just like beef – fat is flavor, so often times the fat found in the fillets or around the belly of the fillet will provide more flavor for that fillet. If you are looking for a more mild taste. or do not particularly like "fishy" flavors on your seafood, you can look for leaner fillets or leaner species in the display case, or talk to your seafood department for their recommendations matching the type of fish you prefer.

Honey

Even honey is graded! But this is a little more confusing and misleading than other forms of grading. Honey grading is not inspected by the FDA or federal inspectors in order to display the USDA grading shield, and displaying the shield is completely voluntary. Honey grading covers Strained Honey, where large particles like honey comb and other natural defects are removed but may still contain pollen, air bubbles and small particles, and Filtered Honey, where the small particles such as air bubbles, pollen and small materials are removed from the honey.

The USDA grading system covers moisture content, absence of defects, flavor, aroma and clarity (for filtered honey). This system, because it is voluntary and does not require an FDA inspection, does not really ensure that the product is graded to any standard and claims can be made about the honey that are untrue. Often the complaint is the honey is watered down or contains additives, added syrups (not from honey) or even containing chemicals and antibiotics.

The grading does not cover these added ingredients, does not verify the floral or botanical source of the honey, does not verify the authenticity of the claims such as raw, unheated, etc. or verify the source, such as country of origin or state of origin. Europe, Australia and New Zealand use a different honey standard when labeling or making claims on honey.

Ultimately the best bet to ensure you are getting the highest quality honey, and that all of the claims on the bottle or jar are 100% accurate, is to know the true source, and to source locally. If you know the farm that is the source of the honey, you can easily determine the accuracy of the claims and choose a higher quality honey that is free from additives such as high fructose corn syrup that do not need to be claimed on packaging.

This honey grading system is calculated on a points system, 100 points is the highest score any honey can get. Some qualities that are used for grading are more objective than others and can make this grading system less standard and uniform in application.

- Grade A
  - Minimum total score of 90 points
  - **Moisture Content** or percent that is water, 18.6% with minimum percent soluble solids at 81.4%
  - **Absence of Defects**, with a score of 37-40, practically free from particles of comb, propolis or other defects that may be deposited in the honey. None of the particles or defect can affect the appearance or edibility of the honey.
  - **Flavor and Aroma** with a score of 45-50 points, a Good score, which means it is free from anything that would negatively impact the taste like smoke, fermentation, outside chemicals or caramelization. The aroma and taste should match that of a floral source.
  - **Clarity** with 8-10 points, meaning the honey is clear and may have air bubbles, pollen or other particles but these are separated and do not take away from the overall appearance of the honey.
- Grade B
  - Minimum total score of 80 points
  - **Moisture Content** 18.6% with minimum percent soluble solids at 81.4%

- ○ **Absence of Defects** with a score of 34-36 points and reasonably free from material deposits that do not affect the appearance or edibility.
- ○ **Flavor and Aroma** score of reasonably good with a score of 40-44 points and is "practically free", meaning it can have traces of smoke, fermentation, outside chemicals, etc. that may negatively impact the overall taste of the honey.
- ○ **Clarity** with 6-7 points and described as reasonably clear with small amounts of materials in the honey suspension that are spaced out without affecting the appearance.
- Grade C
  - ○ Minimum total score of 70 points
  - ○ **Moisture Content** 20% or minimum percent soluble solids at 80%
  - ○ **Absence of Defects** with a score of 31-33 points and fairly free from material defects that do not affect the appearance of edibility.
  - ○ **Flavor and Aroma** with a fairly good score of 35-39 and is reasonably free of contaminants that can cause negative impacts in overall taste.
  - ○ **Clarity** with 4-5 points is fairly clear with more bubbles or pollen in the honey suspension that do not seriously affect the appearance.

Color is not used in the voluntary USDA guidelines used to grade honey; instead, this is more an indication of the strength and flavor of the honey. Dark honeys tend to have stronger flavors than the lighter colored honeys. Sometimes the primary botanical source of the pollen can determine the strength of the honey more than the color can. Linden and Basswood are strong in flavor but light in color while Tulip tree is dark but is a mildly flavored honey.

Raw Honey

Most honey experts and enthusiasts agree that raw honey is of higher quality than the overly filtered and heated alternatives. Raw honey has not been heated above about 95 degrees Fahrenheit (35 degrees Celsius), there are no additives like syrups and there are generally larger occurrences of air bubbles or pollen in the honey solution because it has not been ultra-finely filtered to remove these organic materials that may be present in honey.

Honey is a naturally occurring antibiotic and will not go bad...ever. Raw honeys are generally viewed as worse by those that do not know how to deal with crystallization, which can occur over time, but is not an indication of it going bad or losing taste in any way. Heating honey can cause a breakdown in enzymes that can take away from natural flavors as well as breaking down components like sugars within the honey. Raw honey will crystalize, and to reverse this process, heat to about 100 degrees, by placing the jar in hot water, and stir thoroughly to remove any remaining crystals. The crystalized honey still has all the same health benefits as the liquid honey, the only difference being a sandy texture that may not be desirable in some applications. Only raw honeys will crystalize, so this is a good way to tell if you are really getting what you are paying for.

CHAPTER 6

SANITATION

Sanitation is a hugely important part of agriculture in every aspect, from farms growing produce, rearing livestock, processing facilities, store processing and integrity of the temperature chain. All of these contribute to sanitation and the overall impact this could possibly have on your health, or a potential outbreak of listeria or salmonella. With today's superbugs this is even more important. This is why the USDA is working toward making each ingredient and product 100% traceable; so that the source of the contamination can be found quickly, impacting as few people as possible.

This chapter will briefly look at the practices used from farm to table. However, the focus will be on what you need to look for when shopping in a grocery store, and how your shopping habits may contribute to your overall health and wellbeing. I understand that some may say I sound like I have gone off on a tangent much like a conspiracy theorist. However, this is meant to point out potential issues, not make decisions about what you are willing to risk. Who knows, you might not know that the retailers are playing Russian roulette with your immune system – or it may change purchasing habits for those who have a compromised immune system, while the habits of others will remain unchanged.

Sanitation
Sanitation is often taken for granted, and is usually overlooked by the general public. This chapter will quickly look at some of the standards currently in place for cross contamination and the temperatures that are

important to look for when you are in the store. These may seem like little things – but they can lead to much larger issues. It is important to look out for your health and wellbeing, or the health and wellbeing of others if they have compromised immune systems, so that there is no undue stress to the immune system.

The USDA sets minimum guidelines for sanitation, but every state, county, and city can have additional regulations that change how sanitation is executed in any establishment. I will only cover general guidelines and not specifics, as the specifics are too vast and are always changing. I will also point out some basics that are not law, but will assist you in avoiding any bouts with food-borne illness (commonly referred to as food poisoning).

- Cross Contamination
- Temperatures

Cross Contamination

Cross contamination is when one item comes into contact with another when it should not. You may practice some of these regulations in your own kitchen – for example, keeping everything that will be served raw separated from those foods that will be cooked, and not using the same cutting board for both, unless it is properly washed between uses.

In addition to raw and cooked, you should also practice the same rules when working between species. You should not use the same cutting board, or knife, without properly sanitizing it between species if you are carving a turkey and a ham. If there is a problem on one, failure to clean the knives or cutting boards will cause the bacteria to jump between species, and now everyone is getting sick!

Keep in mind that this is not just limited to your own kitchen – you should look for the same practices being executed at your local grocer and restaurants. Restaurants are much harder to follow unless you are always going to hibachi grills, or other similar restaurants. There is a lot of blind faith that these establishments are following the proper practices. I am not saying not to ever eat out again, but if you see anything, speak up to the server or managers so that it can be fixed; especially if you like the food and want to be able to come back without getting food poisoning.

When it comes to grocers, the easiest way to make sure the practices of sanitation are being properly followed is to watch the deli department; this will usually give you an insight into how the rest of the store operates. Grocers may not have associates that are cross trained throughout the store, and work in all departments, but grocers generally follow the same guidelines throughout their store. You cannot usually see a butcher work or watch as the store cuts fruit, as these are normally done in refrigerated rooms in the back of the store. So watch the deli.

Here is what to watch for:

1. Gloves should be changed when changing species. Does your deli worker change gloves between species when you order Turkey, Deli items, and Salami? It may sound wasteful but there should be three sets of gloves used in order to prevent cross contamination!

2. If gloves are not changed between species, they should at least be changed when switching from meats to cheeses. Does your deli change gloves when you order both meats and cheeses?

3. Fresh cleaning cloths should be available with sanitation water so that messes can be easily wiped up – these cloths should be free of stains, and should be tossed for new ones when stains occur. Using a dirty cloth, or one with visible stains, is no different than mopping a floor with dirty water – all you are doing is moving the bacteria all around the department.

4. Gloves should be changed between hot and cold deli items. These are kept at different temperatures. One is meant to be kept hot, which will lessen the growth of bacteria and at times kill certain strains, and one to be kept cold slowing bacteria growth. Failure to remove gloves or change them between hot and cold

areas in the deli can introduce bacteria from one area to the other. That means the hot bacteria will grow on cold deli items until it has reached the cold temperature, and the cold bacteria will do the same in the new hot environment.

5. Self-grooming should be reserved for the bathroom. When being waited on, you should never see someone, with or without gloves grooming themselves. This means rubbing their face, pulling their ear, smoothing hair, or grooming other regions, and then resuming waiting on someone. There should always be, at a minimum, a change of gloves. Remember, the gloves are there to help stop the spread of germs. By grooming with gloves on, the germs from their face or hair is transferred to the gloves and then to your food. In a perfect world, you should wash your hands before returning with a fresh pair of gloves.

6. Money is filthy! Think of how often you wash your hands before or after handling money, and then how many people have handled that bill. Even credit cards are filthy and should be considered as dirty as money. Cash registers too, they could have food particles, in addition to bacteria from money and credit cards. Anyone handling money should not be handling your food. They should first wash their hands and change gloves. At a minimum, they should change gloves before handling food to keep the germs from the money from transferring to your food.

7. Don't see gloves? This isn't necessarily unsanitary, but the rules of cross contamination are more important to follow, and hands need to be washed more often in order to keep contamination from occurring. Just as with the deli items, it is important that there is no self-grooming or touching services and materials that aren't directly involved in the preparation of food. This is often practiced in kitchens at restaurants; some fast food or deli establishments will allow this, but it is important to watch to ensure that the employees are following proper sanitation practices and not putting anyone at risk. Without easily removable gloves to prevent transfer

of bacteria, hands must be kept clean and washed more often. The washing should occur as often as gloves would be changed.

There are times when an employee will forget to change gloves; they are busy, or there is a long line and they may quickly go through the department without changing gloves at every station. The above points are under ideal conditions. If you feel uncomfortable with the practices for the store in which you shop, ask the management of the department or the store manager if these practices are normal and voice your concerns.

Do not accept excuses. It is usually easy to tell, when you shop frequently at a location, if the practices remain constant and only change around the holidays when everyone is shopping at the same time and long lines may occur. By voicing your concerns with management, you can find out if the retailer is one you are comfortable with, and if they are truly concerned with their customer base.

Insect issues are usually a good indicator of bad sanitation – namely drains. Although commonly annoying bugs like house flies and fruit flies are attracted to rotten fruit, veggies, and meats, they normally do not become an issue because of bad food left out on display tables in grocers. Instead, they are drawn inside due to drain issues. These are most commonly related to the disposal units, and then, once inside, move throughout the building to hover around fruit, veggies, and meats. These insects are hard to get rid of once you have them, but are fairly simple to prevent. If you have them in your house around your fruit bowl, use vinegar traps. Make sure you clean your garbage disposal, clean any liquids from your garbage can, and change your garbage regularly. These insects will soon disappear.

Temperatures

Temperature is important in keeping bacteria and bugs out of food, and keeping the food safe for human consumption. Cool temperatures keep bacteria dormant, so they will not continue to grow and spread. Hot temperatures kill bacteria. Annoying insects that are often found around rotting foods, like fruit flies or common house flies, are often kept away from food with both hot and cold temperatures. Temperatures that are hot enough will burn the fly, much like it would you or me; cold temperatures will actually prevent movement of the fly.

Very cold temperatures, like those in your freezer, will cause the fly to go into a state of hibernation where it may appear dead. Chilled temperatures, like those of your refrigerator or the refrigerated displays you see in your grocer, will prevent the wings from working and the fly is unable to navigate easily. Flies tend to avoid cool temperatures as they like to be able to move. When they are caught they are easy to get rid of and prevent further contamination caused by the fly

Here are some things to keep in mind regarding temperature that you may not have considered:

1. Ice is not meant to bring an item down to a particular temperature; it is only meant to maintain a temperature for a short period of time, around 2 hours, and only then in optimum temperatures below 45 degrees Fahrenheit.
   a. Items that are displayed on ice, should be partially, to mostly, buried in the ice in order to maintain the ideal temperature for items that must be refrigerated.
   b. When displayed outside in high temperatures the ice will melt quickly, and will need to be changed more often. Most states and local regulatory agencies do not allow ice displays outside unless temperatures are below 45 degrees Fahrenheit; otherwise, the temperatures are not being maintained.
   c. A display with mostly water isn't keeping any required temperature, and will make you more at risk of food poisoning if there was any cross contamination or bacteria introduced to the item.

    d. This is especially important for seafood displays, as these cases often place the seafood on top of the ice throughout the day while inside a refrigerated environment. Look for the following indications that the case is not maintaining temperatures, and may potentially make you sick.

        i. Ice should be lose, it should not appear to be a single slab or look like it has melted and then refrozen as a solid piece. This means that the defrost cycle is too long or too hot, and during the melting phase, the bacteria is growing and spreading within the case.

        ii. Ice should appear frozen throughout the case, there should be no standing water in the case; standing water means the ice is not able to remain frozen, and therefore bacteria is growing.

        iii. The case should also be free of debris. If you see scales and pieces of shellfish tails throughout the case, in areas where like scales or shellfish are not being displayed, this often means that the ice is not changed on a regular basis. The debris can contribute to cross contamination, especially when it comes to allergens like shellfish.

    e. Any fruits, vegetables, or meats that have been cut open, and are no longer in their whole state, should be refrigerated; the inside flesh is now exposed to the elements. These items should not be purchased from unrefrigerated displays, or displays that do not have ice to maintain temperatures.

2. Display cases used in retailers often have fill lines that are visible to the customer. They are normally located behind, or below, a shield that is found on a case. When product is found above the shield or above the fill line, the product is not being kept at ideal

temperatures, and will likely not last long in your home. These products could potentially already have bacteria growing. If this is a concern for you, grab one of the packages that is within the fill line indicated on the case.

3. Overfilled display cases are not efficient. For any display case, whether it be in the meat department, deli department, dairy, juices, or cheeses, you should be able to put your hand up around the front of the shelf and feel a slight cool breeze. If you are unable to feel this breeze it means the air flow is blocked. This interruption of air flow will cause items in the front of the case, or closer to the consumer, not to be kept at ideal temperatures.

4. Have you ever heard strange noises out of any display cases? This can often mean that they are running less efficiently, and that temperatures are not being maintained. This is not always true. Some older food cases are just not as efficient as the newer cases that run almost silently. This is usually the case if you are hearing noises you would not normally hear when you are at your favorite grocer.

5. Have you ever noticed a thermometer gage on the outside of the case? This is for the use of the retailer, to monitor the cases to ensure they are keeping temperatures. You can always look at these to see the temperature of the case when you are shopping. If you see a temperature that does not match up with department you are shopping, such as running too high over frozen (32 degrees Fahrenheit) for the frozen department, or too high above room temperature (45 degrees Fahrenheit) for something in a refrigerated section, you can ask questions about the case until you are comfortable that temperatures are being maintained.

CHAPTER 7

EXPIRATION DATE

// **E** xpiration Date" is the date that everyone knows about, or seems to know about, when it comes to food. But what does it really mean, and why are there so many different ways to say the same thing? Is it the same thing? This chapter will look at what some of these different ways to state when something "goes bad" really means. How this affects your health, and how this could impact how you buy in the future.

- Expiration Date
- Sell By Date
- Use By Date
- Best By Date

Expiration Date

This is often used when talking about when something goes bad, but you will not likely see any food items in the store, in any department, that use this wording. This is a general understanding that after a date, something is bad. But, you will see that this is not always the case. The dates you will find on items are determined based on a number of different rationalizations by the companies or corporations releasing the food items. This includes: How long the item is expected to stay on the shelf at the store before being sold, the subsequent length of time the customer will be able to use the product, optimum eating experience (taste, texture, etc.), expected bacterial growth, and if the item is meant to be consumed immediately or if it is expected to sit in a refrigerator for a day or two before use.

All of these determine what date is selected, but not the wording on the product, here is what you will see when you are shopping and what all of this really means.

Sell By Date

This is used primarily on items that are meant to be consumed immediately, or within a short period of time, and will not spend days in a refrigerator before they are consumed. These items are usually labeled by the store; like cut fruit or deli salads that have scale labels. This doesn't mean that the food is bad after this date, just that the store will not have the best reputation if the food does not last after the customer takes it home. In order to keep a good reputation with customers, retailers will shorten the "shelf life" of an item to ensure that when the food gets home it will last more than one day before growing moldy, losing the ideal texture and taste, or starting to smell funny.

Some retailers will make sure that they can get another 2-3 days in sub-optimum conditions. This is equivalent of your own refrigerator. Think of the temperature you have set on your refrigerator, and how often you open and close the door. The inside of the refrigerator is not always maintaining a contestant temperature unless something is shoved way in the back near a vent, so it is important that the items last when they are taken home.

Use By Date

This is usually found on highly perishable items like eggs or bacon, or on your fresh steak from the store. Like sell by dating, this does not refer to safety. This refers to the optimum conditions – best texture, taste, and overall satisfaction for the item. An egg consumed after this date may not look perfect when broken open, and the yolk may appear cloudier than you are used to, if you have never used an egg after the use by date. This does not mean that you are at any risk for consuming an egg that is 2-3 days after the use by date.

Unfortunately, there really isn't a comprehensive list of how long items like meats, eggs, or other items marked with "Use By" dates are good after this date, so best judgements need to be used. Remember, your refrigerator isn't as consistent at keeping temperature as those of a manufacturer or retailers, so experiments conducted in storage will not match your own at home.

Best By Date

Strikingly similar to the above dates, it too refers to the quality, and not safety. This is usually found more on canned goods or boxed items, like boxed dinners or cereals. This means that if the container is unopened, the contents will taste as expected by the manufacturer, and as expected by the customer, up until that date. The product will begin to taste stale, or change texture after this date. This is not the date for open boxes. Open boxes are likely to become infested with moths or other pesky insects if kept until that date while being opened for a long time.

What do you do if it is "expired"?

Some retailers will offer discounts on the day marked on the item, even if it is still good for a few days. By most state laws, items that are expired, by any sell by, use by or best by dating cannot be sold. However, there are some discount grocers or food banks that accept these items and will sell them at large discounts, or in exchange for volunteer work. Items are sold under these conditions because they do not pose a public health risk, they are not curdled or rotting. The dating is used as a guideline to ensure the best experience for the customer, but it doesn't mean the experience will be bad if consumed after the date. However, make sure you are not too far past the date. Even heat pasteurization cannot keep bacteria away forever!

Canned goods past expiration are usually good as long as the can has not been compromised, meaning no denting or bloating. A bloated can should never be opened, this means that bacteria has begun to grow inside the can, usually botulism, and this is potentially deadly.

If you are looking to pinch an extra penny out of your budget, you can begin to keep items after the date on the packaging and see how long it lasts and meets your expectations for taste and overall quality. Make a record of these items so you can shop accordingly, and even get a list of dates so you know when to throw things out or re-date them when you get home. This can even be a time saver, allowing you to go to the store less often because you aren't constantly fighting the dates in your fridge.

> Expiration Dates found on water bottles are for the bottle – not the water! Water doesn't go bad, but bottles used will begin to break down and mix with the water. The water will often look snowy, or like there is salt in the bottle, when this happens.

What About Your Manager's Special?

Some retailers will have "manager's specials", while at times it may mean something different, it usually means that the item is close to expiration or has changed color. These specials are usually used in highly perishable areas where it is important to ensure that product is "turned", or moved out of the department quickly, so that new fresher product can be restocked. Sometimes this means the items are freezer burned if found in the frozen aisles, has turned color (in the case of lunchmeats or other meat items), or is close to the printed date (best by, sell by, or use by) on the package. Just like the dates above, these do not pose a health risk. However, sometimes, either inadvertently, or in order to make a little more money, retailers will mark packages that have become compromised as manager's specials.

In the case of meats, there are a couple of things that can change the color of the meat; temperature change, lights, and oxygen. It is important to check the package to make sure the seals are unbroken and no oxygen has been introduced, and to feel the package to make sure it is cool to the touch. Some types of light can cause meat to turn to a grey or brown color prematurely, and because of the lack of aesthetic appeal, these are usually reduced in price. This type of color change does not pose a health risk, while a change in temperature or a break in the seal does.

This is also true for frozen items. Over time, moisture that was already present in the package will begin to crystalize and create freezer burn, or will begin to change the color and texture of the product. Chicken will usually appear almost transparent, while red meats will start to change to a darker brown color when this happens. It is important to check the package in this case too; if the seals are broken, it means that outside moisture has gotten in to assist in crystallization and freezer burn. This also means that bacteria found its way in too. When the product is defrosted it means that there is more bacteria and a potential health risk to the customer.

CHAPTER 8

WEIGHTS

Tare is something that every customer takes for granted. However, recent headlines have brought this to the attention of many, while it is still not fully understood.

- Tares
- Department of Weights and Measures

The federal government created an agency, the Department of Weights and Measures, to ensure when a claim is made about a weight or volume of something that is sold, the item meets the standards for that weight. Essentially, this department makes sure that the customer isn't shorted or ripped off by retailers. You may be familiar with the silver stickers that are found on grocery market checkout scales showing the month and year of the last inspection for that scale. These scales are locked so that retailers cannot go into them to readjust the calibration, so that they remain accurate. This same sticker is also found on gas pumps to ensure that the displayed dispensed volume of gas matches what you are getting in your tank. Any time you feel that you are being ripped off, you can call your local Department of Weights and Measure, or your local FDA branch to file a complaint and ask for an investigation.

Tare is a term that refers to the weight of the packaging and labeling along with the food in the container. The tare is programmed into scales, either at the point of sale (checkout lane) or in the scales that label the product in the specific department, such as the meat or deli department. The recent headlines regarding overcharging, indicated employees were not programming the tare or were not accounting for the tare before the food was weighed and packaged. This caused the customers to pay extra for packaging.

Retailers are responsible for properly programming and accounting for tare when it applies, and are audited regularly (usually at least once a year) to ensure that they are in compliance in every department. The weights of the packaging materials are normally pre-programmed into the department scales or checkout lanes so that no one has to reset scales. These pre-programmed tares often go in favor of the guests. Have you ever left a store with hot peppers not in a bag from the produce department? This is an item commonly pre-programmed with a tare, without the bag. The tare is subtracted from the total weight of the hot peppers, and the remaining amount is charged to the customer making a very small error in favor of the customer.

Other areas are harder to program. For example, when multiple container sizes or styles are available, or in full-service departments like a full-service meat counter, or a deli department. In this case, you should observe the employees zeroing the scale to the container they will be using, or typing in a known tare before weighing foods. If the scale isn't zeroed out, when the PLU is entered into the scale the scale should initially read a negative number to account for any packaging that is placed on the scale with the food item. If not, you are free to remind the employee to account for the tare.

Some states, like Michigan, have laws that protect the customers and punish the retailers for overcharging or improperly pricing items. This includes not accounting for tare. If you purchase an item and the food item alone doesn't meet the weight on the label, you are entitled to a partial refund, full refund, or an additional fee, depending on local laws. If a retailer gives you a hard time about addressing this issue, feel free to contact the local Department of Weights and Measures.

When an audit is conducted and a retailer is found to be in violation of the Department of Weights and Measures guidelines, and is overcharging or improperly stating weights, they are subject to fines. These are determined based on internal sales data for the items that were found to be in violation, for the predetermined time frame, and the number of locations (in the case of chain stores). If a deli salad was sold, and it was observed or determined that the tare wasn't accounted for in any location for a chain store due to improper training and documentation on the process, and it was found not to be followed for a year, an entire year's sales data on this item would be used to determine the amount of the fine, for every pound or partial pound sold.

CONCLUSION

Food is an industry that is constantly changing. This can be influenced by a number of factors; these include the global economy and overseas policies, how money is spent, and public perception at home. How you spend your money can greatly determine the future of policies, and the direction of future farming and sanitation legislation that is passed in your city or state.

In 2012, the European Union banned a chemical, dimethylnitrosamine (DPA), and in 2015 banned the import of produce that is coated with this chemical. This is a quite common chemical used in the storage of apples to prevent spotting and bruising. Although the chemical itself isn't harmful, it breaks down into chemicals that are carcinogenic. The European Union is now speaking by banning the import of apples from the United States that have DPA – the threshold for tolerance of DPA is less than half in the EU of what it is in the United States.

In 2013 Europe also drove major changes to a famous blue box, yellow-orange pasta. In Europe certain food additives are banned while others may require warnings for consumers. Yellow No. 5, a common food additive in the US requires a label stating "This product may have adverse effect on activity and attentional children." Due to this warning this food coloring has already been removed from European versions of the food, instead using paprika and beta-carotene (used as naturally occurring, non-synthetic colorants). Identical changes have not happened yet for US customers, while only some products within this famous line of pastas will have the food coloring Yellow No. 5 and Yellow No. 6 removed from future versions.

Demand for organic foods has increased in the past few years, rising 11% in just 2014. As more and more is known about the long term impact of GMOs, pesticides, and fertilizers on the environment. The public is speaking up about these concerns by shifting purchasing away from GMO to Organic.

You can make a change and voice your opinion by writing to congress or your senator. The easiest way to get attention about your opinion for better food, organic, grass fed, humanely raised, or local, is to spend your money and buy the foods that mean something to you. By taking your money away from big pharma and large farms, and giving back to your community and naturally or organically raised foods, you are speaking louder than any letter can. Policies won't until you change how you spend your money.

Change can always be made for the better. Take the steps to be informed about your food and the food chain, and to support local farmers and farms with your purchases, so that these positive changes can continue.

REFERENCES

Salmon Nation - Genetically Engineered Salmon?
http://www.salmonnation.com/fish/gefish.html

Survey: Organic Farmers Pay the Price for GMO Contamination
http://www.foodandwaterwatch.org/pressreleases/survey-organic-farmers-pay-the-price-for-gmo-contamination/

Supreme Court: Monsanto Can Sue Farmers Whose Crops Get Inadvertently Contaminated with GMO
http://thefreethoughtproject.com/supreme-court-monsanto-sue-farmers-crops-inadvertently-contaminated-gmo/

5 Reasons High Fructose Corn Syrup Will Kill You
http://drhyman.com/blog/2011/05/13/5-reasons-high-fructose-corn-syrup-will-kill-you/

USDA Agricultural Marketing Service – Standardization Services
http://www.ams.usda.gov/AMSv1.0/sat

Seafood Source – Your Global Seafood Solution
Seafood Handbook: Over 100 Types of Fish & Seafood
www.seafoodsource.com/seafoodhandbook

USDA Agricultural Marketing Service – Country of Origin Labeling
http://www.ams.usda.gov/AMSv1.0/ams.fetchTemplateData.do?temp
late=TemplateM&navID=CountryofOriginLabeling&rightNav1=Count
ryofOriginLabeling&topNav=&leftNav=CommodityAreas&page=Coun
tryOfOriginLabeling&resultType=

Understanding Vaccines: Vaccine Myths Debunked
http://www.publichealth.org/public-awareness/understanding-vaccines/
vaccine-myths-debunked/

Killer Pig Virus Wipes Out More Than 10 Percent of Nation's Hogs,
Causing Spike in Pork Prices
http://www.huffingtonpost.com/2014/04/27/pig-virus-wipes-out-nations-
hogs_n_5221471.html

Miller Amish Poultry
http://millerpoultry.com/

Whole Foods CEOs admit to overcharging, apologize
http://money.cnn.com/2015/07/02/news/companies/whole-foods-
overcharge-apology/

Europe Bans American Apples – Too Toxic to Eat
http://www.globalresearch.ca/europe-bans-american-apples-too-toxic-
to-eat/5387379

Food Business News: U.S. organic food sales rise 11% in 2014
http://www.foodbusinessnews.net/articles/news_home/Consumer_
Trends/2015/04/US_organic_food_sales_rise_11.aspx?ID=%7B0C
1920D3-1822-4467-9FF0-F1EE00E53F54%7D

CNN – Kraft removing artificial dyes from some mac and cheese
http://www.cnn.com/2013/11/01/health/kraft-macaroni-cheese-dyes/

Mother Earth News – The USDA Label Says Grass-fed, but is It?
http://www.motherearthnews.com/homesteading-and-livestock/usda-grass-fed-label-zmaz08amzmcc.aspx

American Grassfed Association – AGA Grassfed Dairy Standards-Draft 06-04-2015-1
http://www.americangrassfed.org/new-aga-grassfed-dairy-standards-open-for-comments/aga-grassfed-dairy-standards-draft-06-4-2015-1/

IFL Science – You can now buy GMO-free water in the U.S.A.
http://www.iflscience.com/chemistry/there-actual-gmo-free-water-sale-us
Honey Traveler – USDA Honey Grading
http://www.honeytraveler.com/types-of-honey/grading-honey/
European Food Information Council – The importance of Omega-3 and Omega-6 Fatty Acids
http://www.eufic.org/article/en/artid/The-importance-of-omega-3-and-omega-6-fatty-acids/Life Extension Magazine – Omega-3 Fatty Acids Increase Brain Volume
http://www.lifeextension.com/Magazine/2010/8/Omega-3-Fatty-Acids-Increase-Brain-Volume/Page-01US Code House Government – 7 USC Ch. 56: Unfair Trade Practices Affecting Producers of Agricultural Products
http://uscode.house.gov/view.xhtml?path=/prelim@title7/chapter56&edition=prelim NPR - Airborne Settles Suit over False Claims
http://www.npr.org/templates/story/story.php?storyId=87937907 Top Class Actions – Judge Trims 5-Hour Energy False Ad. Class Action
http://topclassactions.com/lawsuit-settlements/lawsuit-news/48336-judge-trims-5-hour-energy-false-ad-class-action/ Law 360 – 5-Hour Energy Maker Must Face Deceptive Marketing Suit
http://www.law360.com/articles/446079/5-hour-energy-maker-must-face-deceptive-marketing-suit FDA US Food and Drug Administration: Are Dietary Supplements approved by the FDA?
http://www.fda.gov/AboutFDA/Transparency/Basics/ucm194344.htm

ACKNOWLEDGEMENTS

Special thanks to my mother for helping me make the publication of this book possible and for assistance in the editing process. Thank you to my dad for all of his support and thank you to Corky and Lori Anderson for providing feedback to make this book even better.

Notes

ABOUT THE AUTHOR

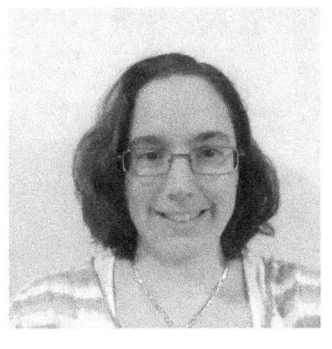 Rachel E. Helwig graduated from Grand Valley State University, in Allendale, Michigan, in 2006. She has worked in the retail grocery industry for over fourteen years in various positions. Rachel's experiences have inspired her to focus on healthy eating while helping others make better eating decisions, and teaching them about foods and health. She is a first-degree black belt in taekwondo and a volunteer at her taekwondo school.

NOTES

NOTES

NOTES